Handbook on
Dental
Materials

**Theory, Multiple Choice Questions, Viva Voce-
Spotters, Model Answers and Practical Exercises
with
48 Colour Plates of Spotter Materials**

Handbook on
Dental
Materials

Theory, Multiple Choice Questions, Viva Voce-Spotters, Model Answers and Practical Exercises
with
48 Colour Plates of Spotter Materials

V Shama Bhat MSc
Professor and Head
Department of Dental Materials
Yenepoya Dental College, Yenepoya University, Mangaluru
Karnataka

Jayaprakash K MSc, PhD
Lecturer
Department of Dental Materials
Yenepoya Dental College, Yenepoya University, Mangaluru
Karnataka

BT Nandish MSc, PhD
Associate Professor
Department of Dental Materials
Yenepoya Dental College, Yenepoya University, Mangaluru
Karnataka

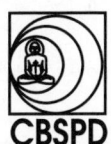

CBSPD

CBS Publishers & Distributors Pvt Ltd

New Delhi • Bengaluru • Chennai • Kochi • Kolkata • Lucknow• Mumbai
Hyderabad • Jharkhand • Nagpur • Patna • Pune • Uttarakhand

Handbook on
Dental
Materials

ISBN: 978-93-86310-86-6

Copyright © Authors and Publisher

First Edition: 2017
Reprint: 2024

Published by Satish Kumar Jain and produced by Varun Jain for

CBS Publishers & Distributors Pvt Ltd
4819/XI Prahlad Street, 24 Ansari Road, Daryaganj, New Delhi 110 002, India.
Ph: 23289259, 23266861   Website: www.cbspd.com   e-mail: delhi@cbspd.com
Corporate Office: 204 FIE, Industrial Area, Patparganj, Delhi 110 092
Ph: 4934 4934   Fax: 4934 4935   e-mail: publishing@cbspd.com; publicity@cbspd.com

Branches

- **Bengaluru:** Seema House 2975, 17th Cross, K.R. Road,
  Banasankari 2nd Stage, Bengaluru 560 070, Karnataka
  Ph: +91-80-26771678/79   Fax: +91-80-26771680   e-mail: bangalore@cbspd.com
- **Chennai:** 7, Subbaraya Street, Shenoy Nagar, Chennai 600 030, Tamil Nadu
  Ph: +91-44-26680620, 26681266   Fax: +91-44-42032115   e-mail: chennai@cbspd.com
- **Kochi:** 42/1325, 1326, Power House Road, Opp KSEB, Ernakulam 682 018,
  Kochi, Kerala, India
  Ph: +91-484-4059061-67   Fax: +91-484-4059065   e-mail: kochi@cbspd.com
- **Kolkata:** 147, Hind Ceramics Compound, 1st Floor, Nilgunj Road, Belghoria,
  Kolkata 700 056, West Bengal, India
  Ph: +91-33-25633055/56   e-mail: kolkata@cbspd.com
- **Lucknow:** Basement, Khushnuma Complex, 7-Meerabai Marg
  (Behind Jawahar Bhawan), Lucknow 226 001, UP, India
  Ph: +0552-4000032   e-mail:tiwari.lucknowi@cbspd.com
- **Mumbai:** PWD Shed. Gala no. 25/26, Ramchandra Bhatt Marg, Next to JJ Hospital
  Gate no. 2, Opp. Union Bank of India, Noorbaug, Mumbai 400 009, Maharashtra, India
  Ph: 022-66661880/89   e-mail: mumbai@cbspd.com

Representatives

• Hyderabad	0-9885175004	• Jharkhand	0-9811541605	• Nagpur	0-8692091830
• Patna	0-9334159340	• Pune	0-9664372571	• Uttarakhand	0-9716462459

Printed at: Rashtriya Printers, Dilshad Garden, Delhi, India

Foreword

It is truly a great privilege and honour to write the foreword for the third consecutive time for my beloved teacher, Prof V Shama Bhat's invaluable attempt in preparing *Handbook on Dental Materials*. The earlier textbook prepared by him, "Science of Dental Materials and Clinical Applications" has no match in our country. It is very fact that, this has been followed and referred extensively in almost all dental schools in this country and abroad, itself speaks volumes about its quality, usefulness and popularity. The third edition, now under print has been revised to keep abreast with the recent developments.

The Science of Dental Materials has become so exhaustive, students in the first and second years of BDS courses, find it extremely difficult to assimilate and reproduce in their examinations. With the vast teaching experience, Prof Bhat, has clearly understood the students' difficulties in facing the theory, viva voce and practical examinations.

To simplify the whole process, he has made an in-depth study of every aspect of the evaluation systems, and with the assistance of his experienced faculty members, BT Nandish and Jayaprakash K (MSc, in Dental Materials with PhD), has provided valuable solutions and answers to all the queries in this subject.

His commitment to this material science (since 1976), is witnessed by visiting the department and its unique museum of materials and models used in dentistry. Inspired by this, Jayaprakash K has contributed another part, large collections of "Skulls and teeth of many domestic animals", which again, is a very unique in our country and elsewhere. We are truly indebted to these invaluable contributions.

I congratulate Prof V Shama Bhat and his supporting staff for these wonderful works which will immensely benefit the students' fraternity and dental profession. I pray Almighty, to shower all His blessings to bestow, Sir (who is very active even at this age of 83 years) with long life and good health for much more contributions in future to the cause of science of dental materials.

BH SRIPATHI RAO MDS
Dean/Principal
Yenepoya Dental College
Mangalore, Karnataka, India
(Former Executive Council Member of DCI
Former Vice-Chancellor, Yenepoya University, Mangalore,
Karnataka)

Preface

Science of materials used in dentistry is a very rapidly advancing composite subject intermeshed by the interaction between the basic science subjects (physics, chemistry, biology) and engineering technologies (polymer resins, metallurgy, ceramics, composites) with the biological sciences (physiology, anatomy, pathology, microbiology, biochemistry). The present scientist–dental clinicians have to select the best materials for the particular clinical situations and apply the highest clinical skills, with the deep knowledge of this very fast developing science. The technicians should have thorough knowledge of metallurgy, ceramics, auxiliary materials, sophisticated pieces of equipment and technologies for selection of best materials and fabrication techniques to avail the desired best properties.

It is said that there is no any dental treatment without using any dental materials in the clinical practices. The importance of the thorough knowledge of this basic science foundation cannot be overstressed. The recent knowledge explosion in the basic sciences, technologies and their clinical applications, has given more responsibilities to the clinicians and technicians. In view of these the Dental Council of India has given the due importance and recently extended the duration of teaching of this subject for two years.

The main objective of the examinations is to evaluate the actual depth of the knowledge of the basic sciences and its applications of the principles acquired during the first two years, which can be later applied scientifically to the treatments in various clinical situations.

The present method of evaluation is, through, theory (long essays, short essays, brief answers, multiple choice questions, and viva voce) and practicals (along with details of answering spotter and questions in memory level).

It is observed, that various types of questions framed such as long essays of about 20 min, short essays of about 10 min, brief answers of about 5 min, durations and also the viva voce methods have their own limitations and are not adequate to assess the actual depth of the knowledge. Candidates are at a loss to plan the extent of information expected within the depth time limit. Recent trend of evaluation of the depth of knowledge of theory, which almost all universities have introduced, is to give more weightages to the multiple choice questions and viva voce examinations. It is quite difficult to answer the viva questions asked at random by the examiners. The spotter and tests, i.e. writing the identifications, compositions, properties and applications of the materials used, as a part of the practical skill tests, actually is a very novel idea which is now followed by all universities.

The Section A contains MCQs, planned for answering the theory and viva voce examination questions, for testing the knowledge in the memory, differentiating and logical levels by using the key answers. In many questions, the three-all correct answers, refer to all the information desired. Much attention is given to provide briefly vast information along with ready reference tables of compositions, properties, etc.

The Section B is focused on the spotter and answers as well as the theory and viva voce examinations. Vast information are provided briefly in nut shell (or capsules!), along with, tables of compositions and properties for quick and ready references. The color plates provided is an additional advantage.

The Section C contains model answers to two university examination question papers. This gives the idea of the contents required to answer the different types of questions within the time limitations—long essays, short essays and brief answers.

The last section comprises a collection of large number of color plates of recent spotter materials for recollection and identifications.

However, there is a lacuna and not much materials and literatures are available in these areas. In view of this, to assist the students and even the faculties, this unique work has been prepared. In addition, model answers to two different University question papers are also provided for the students to practice, planning and answering them in the limited time, by those authors deeply involved in handling this subject (since 1976), as well as writing popular textbooks, "Science of Dental Materials and Clinical Applications", and "Complete solutions to Dental Materials".

V Shama Bhat
Jayaprakash K
BT Nandish

Acknowledgments

The idea of writing this was initiated by Mr Jayaprakash K, Lecturer in DM by collecting large number of color plates and questions for spotters and discussed regarding the details. It took nearly six months to do this work. Dr. BT Nandish Associate Professor, his valuable contributions for preparing this work. Mrs Sowmya Rao, Lecturer, recently joined our department, took active part in this project.

Our thanks are due to our beloved Principal Dr BH Sripathi Rao, Yenepoya Dental College, who has given us continuous support and encouragements, without which we could not have succeeded in any of our endeavors, and development of this department, with the unique museum of materials used in dentistry, and preparing this work.

Our respected Chancellor, Y Abdulla Kunny is always a source of inspirations to all our above adventures, preparing a "Textbook on "Science of Dental Materials and Clinical Applications 3rd Edition (CBS Publishers, 2006)," "Complete Solutions for Dental Materials" questions and answers to many Indian University Question Papers (Jaypee Publishers—2014), this work, as well as developing unique museum of "dental materials, skulls and teeth of animals". We are very much thankful to Dr M Vijayakumar, Vice-Chancellor, Dr CV Raghuveer, Registrar, Dr BT Nandish, Controller of Examinations of our Yenepoya University and all our colleagues for their encouragements.

We sincerely thank Mr SK Jain Managing Director, Mr YN Arjun, Senior Vice President—Publishing, Editorial and Publicity, CBS Publishers & Distributors for readily accepting the manuscripts and bringing out this beautifully planned book in the shortest time possible.

V Shama Bhat
Jayaprakash K
BT Nandish

Contents

Section B

2 Theory–Viva Voce and Spotters

Section C

3 | Theory Model Answers for University Examinations

Practical Curriculum in Dental Materials

Sl. No.	Practical Exercises for First Year
1.	Study of setting action of gypsum products (dental plaster and stone and die stones). Determinations of gloss-disappearance time, initial and final setting times with respect to various water/powder ratios, accelerators, retarders and mixing times using Gilmore needles and Vicat penetrometers. Preparations of regular shaped plaster models trimming and polishing.
2.	Manipulation of impression compound and preparing casts: a. Impression of edentulous die, and regular cast metal dies. b. Preliminary impression of finger with impression compound.
3.	ZnOE impression pastes—mixing and recording secondary impression of the same finger. Preparing finger-cast-duplicate with model or stone plaster.
4.	Manipulation of alginate impression materials: a. Using a cardboard spacer, prepare special tray with impression compound for the metal die, and prepare perforated special tray. b. Record alginate impression of same die. Cover it with wet cotton and prepare the stone cast. c. Recording impression of acrylic partially dentulous die using with alginate and perforated tray and preparing its cast.

5. *Demonstrations:* Manipulation of two consistency elastomers; preliminary impression or tray, secondary, etc. impression techniques, special trays, rubber adhesives, die stone casts.

6. Mixing of heat or cold cure acrylic denture base resin powders with MMA liquids, studying various stages of mixing and dough times.

7. Manipulation of modelling wax and preparation of rectangular block of size 4.0 × 1.2 × 1.0 cm, finishing and polishing of the wax block.

8. *Acrylization:* Wax block is invested, in dental flask and dewaxed. Seperating medium is applied. Heat cure clear acrylic dough is prepared, packed with one or two trial closures, bench-cured for 30 min, cured at 70°C for 8 hr, bench-cooled and recovered. Excess is removed, abraded with 60 and 100 grit sand papers. Polished with pumice and French chalk slurries.

Practical Excercises for Second Year

9. *Manipulation of dental cements:* Selection, proportioning and mixing for luting or base consistencies.

   a. Zinc oxide eugenol cements
   b. Zinc phosphate cements
   c. Zinc polycarboxylate cements
   d. Glass ionomer cement (types I and II).

10. *Demonstrations:* Main instruments, applications of cavity varnishes and liner, cement bases, cement restorations on class 1, 2, 3, 4, 5 tooth cavity models. Luting cements consitencies and cementations.

11. Manipulation of dental amalgam restorative material:

    • Main instruments for mixing mortar and pestles, squeez cloth, amalgam and plastic carriers, round and rectangular condensers, carvers (diamond,

demonstrations, Hollenback's and Wartz's), round and T burnishers, and polishing agents.
- Alloy selection criteria.
- Mercury/alloy ratios, proportioning methods.
- Trituration methods, mulling and squeezing.
- Homogeneous and optimum condensation.
- Carving, burnishing and finishing.

12.	*Demonstrations:* Dental alloy casting procedures: Indirect wax patterns. Spruing methods, casting ring with liners, investing and divesting methods, wax burn out, methods of melting of alloys, casting machines of different types, casting, cooling, devesting, finishing and casting defects.
13.	Demonstrations: Fabrication steps of metal ceramic restoration.
14.	Demonstrations: Fabrication of active and reactive (passive) orthodontic appliances.

Theory, MCQs and Answers

1. Orientation to Dental Sciences

Dentistry is an art of science and clinical skill of applications of recent innovations in science and technologies for preventions, corrections and treatments of health problems of various dental and associated soft and hard tissues, as well as providing desired treatments, permanent oral appliances, many of these being fabricated outside the oral cavity.

1-1. The overriding goal of dentistry is to:
   (a) Maintain or improve the dental health of the patient
   (b) Maintain or improve the clinical skill of the dentist
   (c) Alleviate pain
   (d) Professional gains

1-2. Father of modern dentistry is:
   (a) Dr John Greenwood (Jr.)   (b) Pierre Fauchard
   (c) Phillips Skinner   (d) Dr R Ahmed

1-3. Purpose of studying science of dental materials is to:
   (a) Understand their properties
   (b) Economise cost of the treatment
   (c) Select the best and most appropriate materials
   (d) Manipulate materials quickly

1-4. Dental materials are classified for:
   (a) Arranging them systematically
   (b) Avoiding spurious materials
   (c) Informing the patients the cost of treatment
   (d) Selection of most suitable materials quickly

1-5. Which of the following properties is of least concern for selection of restorative materials?
(a) Biocompatibility   (b) Mechanical properties
(c) Aesthetics   (d) Viscoelasticity

1-6. Match the dental specialities with treatments:

(a) Conservative   (1) Diseases of oral cavities and associated tissues

(b) Prosthodontics   (2) Diseases connected with periodontium

(c) Pedodontics   (3) Prevention and treatments of malocclusions

(d) Orthodontics   (4) Pulpal and periapical pathologies

     (5) Coronal aspects—calcified parts

     (6) All problems of patients of below 14 years

     (7) Fabrications for missing teeth or parts of face

     (8) Educating public and communities

1-7. ADA specifications for dental materials are to:
(a) Reduce the manufacturing cost
(b) Simplify manipulation techniques
(c) Control qualities and standardise testing methods
(d) Standardise the price globally

1-8. The hardest material in the human body is:
(a) Cementum   (b) Femoral bone
(c) Dentin   (d) Tooth enamel

1-9. The densest material in the following (cross-section of tooth):
(a) Acrylic resins   (b) Ceramics
(c) Dentin   (d) Tooth enamel

Properties

(a) Tooth enamel: Very hard, brittle, abrasion resistant, fluorescent, aesthetic, low COTE, good thermal insulator.

Properties, units	Tooth enamel	Tooth dentin	Acrylic teeth	Feldspathic porcelain
Density, gms/cc,	2.97	2.14	1.19	2.5
Proportional limit-(PL), in MPa	224	148	27–45	Low
Compressive strength, CS in MPa	380	300	65–75	170
Tensile strength in MPa	10	51	55–65	25
Young's modulus of elasticity Y = Q = E = MPa	80000	18000	2,500	70,000
Modulus of resilience R = J/m^3	0.55	0.94	0.32	Low
Surface hardness—KHN	340 or 300 VHN	68 or 62 VHN	16–20 Ht. cured	460 or 360 VHN
Thermal conductivity, K = Cals/sec/cm^2/(°C/cm)	0-0022	0.0016	0.006	0.0005
Coefficient of thermal expansion, COTE ppm/°C	11.4	8–6	80—120	9–12
Coefficient of diffusion D = K/sp, heat × density	0.469 mm^2/sec.	0.183 mm^2/sec.		

Table 1.1.1: Approximate properties of human, acrylic and porcelain teeth

(b) **Tooth dentin:** Strong, tough, resilient, opaque, lower COTE, i.e. even better thermal insulator. These protect the pulp, from chemical, electrical, and thermal insults.

(c) **Acrylic teeth:** Common artificial teeth, no roots, Chemically bonds to acrylic denture, high COTE, low abrasive resistance, adequate aesthetic, not expensive.

(d) **Porcelain teeth:** Brittle, abrasion resistant, low COTE, excellent permanent aesthetics, but no chemical bonding and mechanical bonding through rhetoric and diatoric holes and bonding pins, to acrylic denture, produce clicking sound, expensive.

2. Properties of Dental Materials and Some Solved Numerical Problems

Applications of stresses produce proportional elastic and non-elastic deformations in solids depending on their internal structures and rigidities. Liquids also exhibit resistance to deformations (viscosity) and surface energies but cause only permanent deformations. Materials also exhibit visco-elasticity (creep), thermal expansions, conductions, etc. Aesthetics is recognised by Hue, Value, and Chromas.

Deep knowledge of the fundamental properties, their numerical values for evaluations and physical significances are most important to students who become dental clinicians, to clearly understand the behaviours and performances of all materials used in different clinical situations. By this only, one can select the best materials and suitable techniques, most appropriate to the particular clinical situations. With these, dentists can do justice and honour to their most noble sacred profession and become successful scientist-dental clinicians.

2-1. The latent heat of fusion is the heat required to convert unit mass of:
  (a) Solid to liquid at room temperature
  (b) Solid to liquid at its normal transition temperature
  (c) Solid to vapour
  (d) Vapour to solid

2-2. Which of these, is the secondary atomic bond?
  (a) Ionic bond (b) Metallic bond
  (c) Covalent bond (d) Dipole moments

2-3. Metallic bonding is due to:
  (a) Sharing of electrons
  (b) Donation of valency electrons
  (c) Free electrons liberated
  (d) van der Waals' forces

2-4. Most of the metals used for alloying gold are:
  (a) Close packed hexagonal (b) Body centred cubic
  (c) Rhombic (d) Face centred cubic

2-5. Austenitic 18-8 stainless steel has:
  (a) Close packed hexagonal (b) Body centred cubic
  (c) Rhombic (d) Face centred cubic

2-6. Zinc has following type of lattice:
 (a) Close packed hexagonal   (b) Body centred cubic
 (c) Rhombic   (d) Face centred cubic

2-7. Properties of amorphous materials are:
 (a) Do not melt at single melting temperature
 (b) High free electron density
 (c) Constant COTE
 (d) Good conductors of heat and electricity

2-8. Which of the following is not applicable to alloys?
 (a) Ranges of melting temperature
 (b) High free electron density
 (c) Constant COTE
 (d) Opacity

2-9. Which of these are crystalline?
 (a) Casting gold alloys   (b) Ceramics
 (c) Dental waxes   (d) Denture resins

2-10. Stress induced in a body refers to:
 (a) Elastic deformations
 (b) Rigidity
 (c) Internal resistance per unit area
 (d) Deforming force applied per unit area

2-11. Flexure stress refers to:
 (a) Compression   (b) Tensile
 (c) Shear   (d) All of the above

2-12. Stress of one MPa is equal to:
 (a) 145 Psi   (b) Newton meters
 (c) 10 Newton/meters^2 (d) Kgm per cm^2

2-13. Strain is expressed in:
 (a) Poise   (b) Pascals
 (c) cms/sec   (d) None of the above

2-14. Proportional limit refers to:
 (a) Maximum stress in straight line part of stress-strain graph
 (b) Maximum strain recovering completely
 (c) Maximum stress relaxation
 (d) Maximum energy absorbed before fracture

2-15. Flexibility or elastic range refers to the maximum:
(a) Maximum stress of stress-strain graph
(b) Strain recovering completely
(c) Energy required fracturing relaxation
(d) Energy absorbed before fracture

2-16. Tensile strength of high copper silver amalgam in MPa is:
(a) 10–12
(b) 68
(c) 138
(d) 2100

2-17. Yield strength of beta titanium (in MPa) is:
(a) 230
(b) 430
(c) 930
(d) 1,630

2-18. Compressive strength of $ZnPO_4$ cement base in MPa is:
(a) >35
(b) >75
(c) >103
(d) >230

2-19. Modulus of resilience is defined as:
(a) Work required to fracture the material
(b) Rigidity or flexibility of material
(c) Thermal energy absorbed per unit volume/°C
(d) Energy stored per unit volume when stretched up to PL

2-20. Modulus of resilience of tooth dentin, in J/m^3, is:
(a) 0.5
(b) 0.9
(c) 12.6
(d) 37.8

2-21. Match the following terms of the stress-strain graph:
(a) Slope within proportional limit
(b) Area up to PL with strain axis
(c) Total area up to fracture
(d) Strain at proportional limit
(e) Stress for 0.2% permanent strain.

(1) Flexibility
(2) Toughness/brittleness
(3) Modulus of elasticity
(4) Yield strength
(5) Fracture resistance
(6) Elastic range
(7) Ultimate strength
(8) Modulus of resilience
(9) Poisons' ratio

2-22. Match the modulus of elasticities (in MPa) of materials:

(a) Chromium-cobalt alloys	(1) 2,450
(b) Tooth dentin	(2) 14,000
(c) Denture-resins	(3) 41,000
(d) Nickel-titanium alloy	(4) 71,000
(e) 18–8 stainless steel	(5) 110,000
(f) Gold alloys	(6) 160,000
	(7) 200,000
	(8) 220,000
	(9) 330,000

2-23. Punch or push-out testing method is used to find:
  (a) Compressive strength
  (b) Tensile strength
  (c) Shear strength
  (d) Flexure strengths

2-24. Tear strength of elastomers approximately (in gm/cm) is about:
  (a) 400   (b) 800
  (c) 1,240   (d) 2,600

2-25. Elastic recovery of additional polysilicone impression is:
  (a) 93%   (b) 97.5%
  (c) 98%   (d) 99.93%

2-26. Dynamic impact strength is measured by using:
  (a) Izod or Charpy testers
  (b) Universal testing machine
  (c) Interferometers
  (d) Three or four point bending test methods

Note: Impact strengths of, tooth enamel = 0.7–1.3, dentin = 3.1, feldspathic porcelain = 0.75, composite resins = 0.8–2.5, stabilised zirconia = 8 in MPa-m$^{\frac{1}{2}}$, respectively.

2-27. Advantages of Knoop's hardness testing method is:
  (a) Micro-surface hardness with minimum indentation
  (b) Used for all hard and brittle dental materials
  (c) Used for elastically recovering ductile or malleable materials
  (d) All of the above

2-28. **Match the surface hardness (in KHN) of the following:**
(a) Denture acrylic teeth resins   (1) 18–20   (2) 55–60
(b) Glass ionomer cement   (3) 68–70   (4) 110
(c) Tooth enamel   (5) 345   (6) 500
(d) Quartz-sand abrasive   (7) 800   (8) 2,500
(e) Carbide-burs   (9) 10,000

2-29. **Surface hardness of elastomers and rubbers are compared by:**
(a) Vicat Penetrometer
(b) Shore-A durometer
(c) Kreb's penetrometer
(d) Reciprocating rheometer

2-30. **Low surface tension and angle of contacts of liquids:**
(a) Prevent wetting of solid surfaces
(b) Cause wetting and used as detergents
(c) Increase setting times
(d) None of the above

2-31. **Surface tension of saliva at 37°C, in dynes/cm is about:**
(a) 45–55   (b) 68–72
(c) 435   (d) 1100

2-32. **Surface tension reducing (wetting) agent is applied on:**
(a) Wax patterns before investing
(b) Stone casts before preparing record base
(c) Tube–impression before electroforming
(d) Glass ionomer cement immediately after restoration

2-33. **Time dependent deformations (creep) and incomplete elastic recoveries by stress relaxations refer to:**
(a) Highly viscous fluids
(b) Newtonian liquids
(c) Pseudoplastic materials
(d) Viscoelastic materials

2-34. **Viscosity of pseudoplastic materials:**
(a) Increases at higher shear rate
(b) Increases at higher compression
(c) Decreases at higher shear rate
(d) Remains constant

2-35. Consistency of $ZnPO_4$ luting cement (under 125 gms load) is:
(a) 20–25 mm
(b) 30–35 mm
(c) 75 mm
(d) 103 mm

2-36. Consistency of type one, ZnOE impression paste mix-held under 500 gm load for 10 min:
(a) 20–30 mm
(b) 30–35 mm
(c) 35–55 mm
(d) 60–65 mm

2-37. Coefficient of thermal expansion should be very large for:
(a) Impression materials
(b) Tooth restorative materials
(c) Solders and brazers
(d) Investment materials

2-38. COTE. of tooth enamel in ppm/°C is:
(a) 8.6
(b) 11.4
(c) 25
(d) 80–120

2-39. Coefficient of thermal conduction should be high for
(a) Impression materials
(b) Tooth restorative materials
(c) Cement bases
(d) Pit and fissure sealants

2-40. Coefficient of thermal conduction of tooth dentin in cg units is:
(a) 8.6
(b) 0.006
(c) 0.0022
(d) 0.0016

2-41. Primary colours in visible light are:
(a) Red, green and blue
(b) Yellow, cyan and magenta
(c) Ultraviolet and infrared
(d) Violet, yellow and orange

2-42. Colour parameter chroma refers to:
(a) Dominant wave-lengths
(b) Intensity or brightness of illumination
(c) Colour saturation
(d) Nature of light emitting source

2-43. Tristimuli colour parameters are measured by using:
(a) Colorimeters
(b) Optical densitometers
(b) Turbidy meters
(d) Munsell's colour system

2-44. Colour-matching of restorative materials with tooth, cannot be done perfectly, since:
(a) Light is electro-magnetic radiation in nature
(b) Light of particular source has wave-length ranges
(c) Enamel is optically anisotropic, i.e. HVC values are different at different points and directions for different wave-lengths
(d) Materials of suitable shades are not available

Solve the following problems to clearly understand the physical properties

P-1. Biting force of 50 kgm acts on the first molar tooth cusp of 2 square mm area. Calculate the stress produced

Solution

Stress = F/A = 50×9.8 N/2×10^{-6} = 245×10^6 Pa. = **245 MPa**

P-2. Calculate the tensile force required to break 18–8 stainless steel orthodontic wire of 0.4 mm diameter (given UTS = 2,100 MPa).

Solution

UTS = F/A, i.e., Force (F) = UTS × Area = UTS · πr^2
$= 2100 \times 10^6 \times \pi r^2 = 2100 \times 10^6 \times 3.14 (0.2 \times 10^{-3})^2$
$= 2100 \times 3.14 \times 0.04$
$2100 \times \pi r^2$ = **263.76 N** = 263.76×0.102 **kgf** = **27 kgf.**

P-3. A wire of two meters length, 0.4 mm diameter, when stretched by 20 kgm load elongates by 16 mm (which is max. elastic recovery). Calculate the stress (proportional limit), strain and modulus of elasticity. If the yield load is 20.3 kgm, find its yield strength, flexibility, and modulus of resilience.

Solution

PL = stress = $\mathbf{20} \times 9.8$ N/πr^2 =
$20 \times 9.8/\pi \times (0.2/1000)^2$N/m^2 = **1560 MPa**

Yield stress = $\mathbf{20.3} \times 9.8$ N/πr^2 =
$20 \times 9.8/\pi \times (0.2/1000)^2$N/m = **2,028 MPa**

Max recoverable strain = Elastic range = flexibility =
0.016/2 = 0.008.

Modulus of elasticity = stress/strain, = P.L./0.008 =
1560/0.008 MPa

= 195,000 MPa (18-8 stainless steel?)

Modulus of resilience = $P^2/2E$ = 1560 × 1560/2 × 195000
= 6.24 J/m³

P-4. A Nittinol orthodontic wire of square cross-section, and thickness, 0.5 mm has modulus of elasticity = 41,000 MPa, Yield strength = 430 MPa calculate elastic range, modulus of resilience, and springiness.

Solution

Elastic range = flexibility (strain) =
= YS/E, = 430/41000 = **0.0104.**

Modulus of resilience = $(YS)^2/2E$ = **2.233 J/m³.**

Springiness = strain/stress = 1/E = 1/41,000 MPa **= 2.4 × 10⁻⁵/MPa**

P-5. A cylindrical sample of silver amalgam, 8 mm length and 4 mm diameter was prepared and preserved at 37°C, for 1 week. When it was stressed by 36N for 1 hour and 4 hrs, the heights decreased to 7.771 and 7.769 mm. Calculate the creep in 3 hrs.

Solution

Creep = $(h_1 - h_2) × 100/h_1$ = (7.771–7.769)100/8 **= 0.025%.**

P-6. Water at 30°C., rises to a vertical height of 2.8 cm in a glass tube of 1.0 mm capillary diameter. Calculate surface tension of water, given, g = 980 cm/sec², angle of contact = 0, d = 1 gm/cc)

Solution

Surface tension at 30°C = hrdg/2 Cos θ = 2.8 ×
0.05 × 1.0 × 980/2 = **68.6 dynes/cm.**

P-7. Weight of 50 drops of saliva falling freely from a vertical glass tube of external diameter 3.6 mm is 1.6 gm. Calculate surface tension of saliva.

Solution

Surface tension = mg/3.8r, (where,m = 1.6/50 = 0.032 gms and g = 980 cm/sec²). = 0.032 × 980/3.8 × 0.18 **= 45.8 dynes/cm.**

P-8. Calculate the force required to dislodge vertically, a complete denture having tissue contact area (A) = 14 square cm, ST of saliva = 48 dynes/cm, assume angles of contacts of saliva with denture and oral tissues, 75 and 55 degrees respectively and average saliva film thickness (t) as 0.2 mm

Solution

Force acting = AT (Cos θ_1 + Cos θ_2)/t =

= 14 × 48 (Cos 75 + Cos 55)/0.02 = 33600 (0.2588 + 0.3548)

= 33600 × 0.6136 = **20617 dynes**.

P-9. A pellet of PBM alloy has volume, 2 cc., sp, gravity = 8.35, sp. heat = 0.21, and latent heat of fusion = 75 cals/gm. Calculate the heat required to heat it from 30° to 1250°C and then melt it.

Solution

Heat required to heat up to 1250°C,

= m × s × (T_1-T_2) Cals. = 2.0 × 8.35 × 0.21 × 1220 = **4,000 cals.**

Heat required to melt = mL = 2.0 × 8.35 × 75 = **1247 cals.**

Total amount heat required = **5247 cals.**

P-10. Calculate the % shrinkage of an impression compound impression of 3 mm. thickness, when cooled to room temperature, 27°C. Given, COTE of impression compound = 320 ppm/°C.

Solution

COTE = 320 × 10^{-6} = (D-d)/D(37°C–27°C).

Shrinkage = (D-d) = 320 × 10^{-6} × 10 × 3 mm = **0.096 mm.**

Percentage shrinkage = 0.096 × 100/3 = **3.2%**

P-11. The lengths of PBM alloy sample are 20 cm and 20.02 cm at 30°C and 100°C. Calculate its COTE.

Solution

COTE. = L_2–L_1/(100–30) × L_1 = 0.02/70 × 20,

= .02/1400 = **14.3 × 10^{-6}/°C. = 14.3 ppm/°C.**

P-12. A solid cylinder of copper of 6 cm diameter and 20 cm length is kept in contact with a steam chamber at one end and a block of ice at the other end. If 95 gm of ice melts/min, calculate thermal conductivity of copper. (Latent heats of steam and ice are 540 and 80 cals/gm respectively)

Solution

Quantity of heat flowing per sec, $Q/t = K.A\ (T_1-T_2)/D$. Cal/sec

i.e. $95 \times 80/60 = K \cdot \pi(3)^2 \times (100-0)/20$. Cals/sec

K = 0.9 cals/sec/cm²/unit temperature gradient.

P-13. Calculate the heat flowing per sec, through 8 mm² area of $ZnPO_4$ cement base of one mm thickness when the temperature of the silver amalgam restoration in contact (with hot beverage), rises to 45°C, K of $ZnPO_4$ is 0.003 Cals/sec/cm²/ unit temperature gradient.

Solution

Heat flowing/sec = $KA(T_1-T_2)/d$ cals/sec

= $0.003 \times 0.08(45-37)/0.1$ = **0.0192 cals/sec**

P-14. 58 gm of water flows in 10 min through a horizontal capillary tube of 1 mm diameter and 50 cm length, under a constant pressure exerted by water of 20 cm height. Calculate the coefficient of viscosity of water.

Solution

Mass of water flowing in 10 min = m = $P\pi\ r^4 t/8l\eta$. (P = hdg).

Coefft. of viscosity = $\eta = P\pi\ r^4 t/8l\ m$ =

$20 \times 1 \times 980 \cdot \pi\ (0.05)^4 \times 600/8 \times 50 \times 58$ Poise = 0.01 Poise = **1 Cp.**

P-15. An elastomeric impression has elastic recovery, 99.92%, polymerisation shrinkage (linear), 0.02% and COTE = 165 ppm/ °C. Calculate the total percentage dimensional change when the impression is brought down to 27°C.

Solution:

Thermal contraction − (COTE) × (T_1-T_2) × 100%

= $165 \times 10^{-6} (37-27) \times 100\%$ = 0.165%.

Total linear shrinkage = Polymerisation shrinkage + incomplete elastic recovery + thermal shrinkages = 0.02 + 0.08 + 0.165 = **0.265%.**

3. Impression Materials

These are elastic and non-elastic materials, carried to the mouth in the unset semi-fluid state, which on setting, should give accurate negative reproduction of the finer details of the oral tissues without any dimensional changes.

3-1. Impression materials should be highly elastic for:
(a) Dimensional accuracy
(b) Easy manipulation
(c) Prevention of tearing while dislodging
(d) Withdrawing thro' severe undercuts

3-2. For obtaining minimum dimensional change, impression materials should have:
(a) Minimum COTE.
(b) Complete elastic recovery
(c) No setting expansion or contraction
(d) All of the above

3-3. Classification of impression materials is done for:
(a) Assessing the properties
(b) Estimating the cost of treatment
(c) Selection of desired instruments
(d) Selection of the best material, most suitable for the particular clinical conditions, quickly

3-4. Zinc oxide eugenol impression material is classified as:
(a) Nonelastic, muco-static, chemically setting
(b) Thermoplastic, muco-compressive, physically setting
(c) Elastic, thermo-setting, muco-static, reversible
(d) Elastic, chemically setting, muco-compressive

3-5. Advantages of special trays:
(a) Uniform thin section of impressions
(b) Less distortion and dimensional changes
(c) Less wastage
(d) All of the above

3-6. Disadvantages of metal stock trays:
(a) Non uniform thick impression causing distortion of impressions
(b) Sterilization is required
(c) More material is required
(d) All the of above

3-7. Rim-lock impression trays are used for:
(a) Agar-agar   (b) Zinc-oxide eugenol
(c) Impression compound   (d) Elastomers

3-8. Oils, fats, stearic acids in impression compounds:
(a) Act as fillers to strengthen
(b) Contribute thermoplastic properties
(c) Plasticizers to control flow
(d) To impart colours

3-9. Flow of type one impression compound at 46°C, as per ADA specifications, should be:
(a) >85% (b) 75–85%
(c) < 6% (d) <2%

3-10. Last portion of the impression compound to harden is, at the:
(a) Tissue surface (b) Within the impression
(c) Simultaneously (d) Tray contact surface

3-11. Disadvantages of impression compounds is:
(a) Its cost
(b) Thermoplasticity
(c) Manipulation technique
(d) Flow and muco-compressive properties

3-12. Green stick compound is used for:
(a) Border moulding, tracing
(b) Secondary impressions
(c) Functional impressions
(d) Cleft-palate impressions

3-13. ZnOE impression material is:
(a) Chemically setting (b) Thermoplastic
(c) Muco-compressive (d) Elastic

3-14. Accelerators of ZnOE impression material is:
(a) $CaCl_2$ and moisture
(b) Mineral or vegetable inert oils
(c) Lower temperatures above dew point
(d) Borax and borates

3-15. ZnOE impression material sets by:
(a) Chelate reaction
(b) Acid–base reaction
(c) Only in presence of moisture
(d) All of the above

3-16. Initial setting-time of type one ZnOE impression material is:
(a) 3–6 min
(b) <10 min
(c) 8–12 min
(d) <15 min

3-17. Hardness of ZnOE impression material is found by:
(a) Vicat penetrometer
(b) Shore-A durometer
(c) Gilmore needles
(d) Krebs penetrometer

3-18. Type-one ZnOE impression material is classified as:
(a) Soft set
(b) Hard set
(c) Thicker consistency
(d) Slow setting

3-18A. Type-two ZnOE impression material is classified as:
(a) Soft set
(b) Slow setting
(c) Thicker consistency
(d) All of the above

3-19. Modifications of ZnOE impression material is done due to:
(a) Burning sensation
(b) Allergic reactions
(c) Special trays required
(d) All of the above

3-20. Properties of hydrocolloid-gels are:
(a) Syneresis and imbibitions
(b) Dependence on rate of loading
(c) Low tensile and tear strengths
(d) All of the above

3-21. Agar-agar impression material contains borax to:
(a) Lower the viscosity
(b) Increase density of brush-heaps and strength
(c) Lower the gelation temperature
(d) Reduce gelation time

3-22. Elastic recovery of agar-agar impressions is about:
(a) 95%
(b) 97.5%
(c) 99%
(d) 99.93%

3-23. Grainy surface of agar-agar impressions is due to:
(a) Inadequate boiling of gel
(b) Low storage temperature
(c) Prolonged storage time
(d) All of the above

3-24. Alginate impression material-powder contains soluble salts of K, Na, or NH_4 alginates, about:
(a) 2–3%
(b) 7%
(c) 15–16%
(d) 50–60%

3-25. Accelerator in alginate impression powder is:
(a) Na_3PO_4
(b) $CaSO_4$
(c) K-Ti-Fluoride
(d) Diatomaceous earth

3-26. Na_3PO_4 in alginate impression powder acts as:
(a) Gelation delayer
(b) Filler
(c) Gelation reactor
(d) Accelerator

3-27. Normal setting alginate impressions has setting times:
(a) 2–4 min
(b) 5–6 min
(c) <10 min
(d) < 15 min

3-28. Compressive-gel strength of alginate should be more than:
(a) 0.343 MPa
(b) 2.4 MPa
(c) 2.5 MPa
(d) 700 gms/cm

3-29. If tear strength of alginate impression is 800 gm/cm, the force required to tear impression of 4 mm thickness is – in grams:
(a) 200
(b) 320
(c) 640
(d) 3200

3-30. Syneresis of alginate impression causes:
(a) Contraction
(b) Expansion
(c) Decrease of strength
(d) Decrease of hardness

3-31. The alginate impression should be dislodged by single sudden jerk to get:
(a) Higher mechanical properties
(b) Minimum distortions
(c) Larger elastic recoveries
(d) All of the above

3-32. Cast should be prepared immediately in alginate impression to:
(a) Save time of technician
(b) Have minimum dimensional change
(c) Get maximum strength of cast
(d) Have none of these

3-33. Laminate technique is used for alginate impression with:
(a) Light-body elastomer
(b) Regular body elastomer
(c) Zinc oxide eugenol
(d) Agar-agar

3-34. Modified dust free alginate (DFA) contains:
(a) Glycerine or glycol   (b) Silicone polymers
(c) Disinfectants   (d) No strengthening fillers

3-35. Tearing of alginate impressions is due to:
(a) Inadequate thickness
(b) Premature removal
(c) In homogeneous and prolonged mixing
(d) All of the above

3-36. Distortion of alginate impression is due to:
(a) Movement of tray during gelation
(b) Premature removal
(c) Delay in pouring the cast
(d) All of the above

3-37. ADA specification for duplicating materials:
(a) Permanent deformation < 3%
(b) Tear strength >900 gm/cm
(c) Strain in compression 4–25%
(d) All of the above

3-38. Elastomeric impression materials have:
(a) Short chained polymer structures
(b) Highly cross-linked structures
(c) Limited cross-linked, coiled, long chained structures
(d) All of the above

3-39. Amount of fillers in regular body (medium consistency) elastomeric impression materials is about:
(a) 15%   (b) 25%
(c) 35%   (d) 55–65%

3-40. Reactor in condensation type polysilicone elastomeric impression materials is:
(a) Lead peroxide   (b) Ethyl silicate
(c) Poly di-methyl vinyl silane   (d) Sulphonic acid

3-41. The usual catalyst in addition-polysilicone impression material is:

(a) Alkyl benzoate   (b) Potassium sulphate

(c) Chloro-platinic acid   (d) Tin octovate

3-42. Addition polysilicone impression material has least:

(a) Dimensional changes in 24 hrs

(b) Percentage flow

(c) Incomplete elastic recovery (permanent deformation)

(d) All of the above

3-43. The by-product during setting of polysulphide impression material is:

(a) Water   (b) Ammonia

(c) Hydrogen sulphide   (d) None

3-44. Main drawback of poly sulphide impression material is:

(a) COTE   (b) Disagreeable odour

(c) Tear resistance   (d) Flexibility

3-45. The by-products in condensation polysilicone impression material is:

(a) Water   (b) Ammonia

(c) Hydrogen sulphide   (d) C_2H_5OH

3-46. COTE of elastomeric impression materials in ppm/°C are about:

(a) 11.4   (b) 25–50

(c) 150–225   (d) 310–550

3-47. Tear strengths of elastomers (in gm/cm) are about:

(a) 200–300   (b) 400–600

(c) 800–940   (d) 2200–3200

3-48. Causes for dimensional changes of elastomeric impression materials:

(a) Thermal contractions

(b) Polymerisation shrinkage

(c) Incomplete elastic recovery

(d) All of the above

3-49. Plasticizer in poly ether impression material is:
(a) Dibutyl phthalate   (b) Glycol ether phthalate
(c) Colloidal silica   (d) Stearic or palmetic acids

3-50. Tray adhesive used for elastomeric impression materials is:
(a) Butyl rubber or styrene dissolved in ketone or chloroform
(b) Methyl methacrylate monomer
(c) Vinyl silane
(d) None of these

3-51. Syringe type light body elastomer is used for:
(a) Double mix double impression technique only
(b) Double mix single impression technique only
(c) Both the above (a) and (b) techniques
(d) Monophase-pseudoplastic materials

3-52. Causes for distortion of elastomeric impressions:
(a) Incorporation of moisture during mixing
(b) Incomplete polymerisation
(c) Too thick and non uniform impressions
(d) All of the above

3-53. Which is NOT used as duplicating material?
(a) Agar-agar
(b) Addl. polysilicone
(c) Alginates
(d) ZnOE

3-54. The setting times of elastomers is determined by:
(a) Gilmore needles
(b) Reciprocating rheometer
(c) Krebs penetrometer
(d) Interferometer

3-55. Impression technique for monophase pseudoplastic elastomeric impressions is:
(a) Double mix-single impression
(b) Double mix-double impression
(c) Reline
(d) Single mix-single impression

4. Gypsum Products (Auxiliary Materials)

Most of the oral appliances require high temperatures for fabrication and they are to be prepared outside the oral cavities. For this their dimensionally accurate, hard positive replicas (dies and casts) are needed using auxiliary materials.

4-1. Chemical formula for gypsum products used in dentistry is:
(a) $CaSO_4$ (b) $CaSO_4 \frac{1}{2} H_2O$
(c) $CaSO_4H_2O$ (d) $CaSO_4 .2H_2O$

4-2. Dental stone is manufactured by:
(a) Fritting   (b) Sintering
(c) Dry calcinations   (d) Autoclaving

4-3. Lattice structure of calcium sulphate hemihydrates is:
(a) Simple cubic   (b) Hexagonal
(c) Orthorhombic   (d) Monoclinic

4-4. Approximate W/P for dental stone is:
(a) 18.6%   (b) 30%
(c) 53%   (d) 60%

4-5. Gilmore needles are used to measure:
(a) Setting times   (b) Setting expansions
(c) Compressive strengths   (d) Surface hardness

4-6. Vicat needle measures setting time by:
(a) Indentation   (b) Penetration
(c) Gloss disappearance   (d) Compression

4-7. Setting times of dental stone, as per ADA specifications-25, in minutes are:
(a) 4 ± 1 (b) 8 ± 2
(c) 12 ± 4 (d) 16 ± 6

4-8. The suitable best accelerator for setting of gypsum products is:
(a) K_2SO_4 (b) $NaCl > 6\%$
(c) Borax   (d) $CaCl_2$

4-9. Setting time of gypsum products is decreased by:
(a) Hot water   (b) Cold water
(c) More water   (d) Mixing for longer time

4-10. **To increase working time and decrease setting times of gypsum products, add:**
(a) Accelerator   (b) Retarders
(c) Accelerator + retarder   (b) More water

4-11. **Maximum setting expansion of type 1V dye stone is:**
(a) 0.1%   (b) 0.15%
(c) 0.2%   (d) 0.3%

4-12. **Normal setting expansion is decreased by:**
(a) Accelerators
(b) Retarders
(c) More water
(d) Any of these

4-13. **Hygroscopic setting expansion (HSE) is increased by using:**
(a) Extra water after initial set
(b) High water powder ratio
(c) Chemical accelerators
(d) Borax

4-14. **Minimum wet (1 hr) strength of dental stone, in MPa is:**
(a) 9   (b) 20.7
(c) 34.5   (d) 48.3

4-15. **Compressive strength of gypsum products is increased by:**
(a) Lower W/P   (b) Longer or faster mixing
(c) Accelerators   (d) Borax

4.16. **Main consideration for selection of dye materials is:**
(a) Biocompatibility
(b) Cost
(c) Thermal expansion
(d) Strength, dimensional stability and hardness

4-17. **Most common die material used in dentistry is:**
(a) Type-3 gypsum product
(b) Type-4 gypsum product
(c) Ceramics
(d) Silver amalgam

4-18. **Metalizing agent used for copper electroforming of dies is:**

(a) Silver dust   (b) Platinum foil

(c) Gold foil   (d) Copper dust

4-19. **Electroformed dies with silver are not prepared due to:**

(a) High cost of silver   (b) Toxicity of silver

(c) Toxicity of electrolyte   (d) None of these

5. Dental Polymer Resins

Clear basic knowledge of the fundamentals of different types of polymerisations of many resin polymers used in dentistry and in almost all other areas in industries or daily life, is a must to select most suitable material and techniques.

5-1. **Which of the following is not a naturally occurring polymer?**

(a) Cotton   (b) Silk

(c) Rubbers   (d) Denture resin

5-2. **Monomer refers to:**

(a) Single reacting chemical unit

(b) Simple polar molecule

(c) Single polymer chain

(d) Oligomer

5-3. **Physical state of polymer may be:**

(a) Flexible-fibrous   (b) Rigid solid

(c) Liquid   (d) Any one

5-4. **Polymerisation of monomers can be initiated by free radicals, produced from chemicals activated by:**

(a) Heat   (b) Chemicals

(c) UV or visible light   (d) Any one

5-5. **Degree of polymerisation refers to:**

(a) Polymerising temperature

(b) Amount of cross-linking

(c) Ratio of average mol. weight of polymer and mol. weight of monomer

(d) Percentage of elasticity or plasticity

5-6. Common cross-linking agent used in acrylic resins is:
(a) Benzoyl peroxide
(b) Dimethyl para toluidine
(c) Dibutyl phthalate
(d) Glycol dimethacrylate

5-7. Example for step growth polymerisation is:
(a) Polysulphides elastomers
(b) Poly methyl methacrylate denture base materials
(c) Polyethers
(d) Polystyrenes

5-8. Camphoro-quinone is used as initiator of poly-merization of resins activated by:
(a) Visible light   (b) UV rays
(c) Thermal energy   (d) Chemical energy

5-9. Termination of polymerisation is by:
(a) Collision with a free radical or another growing polymer
(b) Exhaustion of all monomers
(c) Chain-hydrogen ion transfer
(d) Any of the above

5-10. Which property does NOT apply to addition-polymers?
(a) Rapid polymerisation
(b) Same chemical properties but different physical properties of monomers
(c) Mol. wt. of polymer = sum of mol. wts of all monomers
(d) Low degree of polymerisation

5-11. Property of thermo-set polymers is:
(a) On heating they soften or melt
(b) Decompose at high temperatures
(c) Low impact strength
(d) Soluble in organic solvents

5-12. Thermoplastic resins soften at higher temperatures (Tg). if:
(a) Degree of polymerisation is lower
(b) More plasticizers are added
(c) Cross-linking is higher
(d) Copolymers with long pendent-side chains

5-13. Internal or external plasticizers are used to increase:
   (a) Rigidity   (b) Surface hardness
   (c) Flexibility   (d) Glass-transition temperature

6. Prosthetic Applications of Polymer Resins

Complete denture is a removable dental prosthesis (oral appliance) that replaces the entire dentition and associated structures of the maxilla and mandible. This contains artificial teeth attached to the denture base which is supported through the contact with underlying oral tissues. Partial denture can be defined as a removable dental prosthesis that replaces missing teeth and associated tissues.

These should serve the main functions of mastication and aesthetic harmony, withstanding all the fluctuating hostile environments of oral cavity such as temperatures, acidities, large dynamic masticating forces, etc.

6-1. Biological requirements of denture base materials are:
   (a) Biocompatibility
   (b) Noncarcinogenic, nontoxic
   (c) Chemically inert and resist chemical attacks
   (d) All of the above

6-2. Denture materials should have high strength to resist:
   (a) Abrasions   (b) Deformations
   (c) Fractures   (d) Creep

6-3. Denture materials should have high modulus of elasticity to resist:
   (a) Abrasions   (b) Deformations
   (c) Fractures   (d) Creep

6-4. Denture materials should have high resilience to resist:
   (a) Abrasions
   (b) Deformations
   (c) Absorption of masticating energies
   (d) Diffusion of heat

6-5. Denture materials should have high surface hardness to resist:
   (a) Abrasions   (b) Deformations
   (c) Absorption of masticating energies (d) Creep

6-6. Denture materials should have low COTE for:
(a) Relishing hotness, taste   (b) Resist softening
(c) Dimensional stability   (d) Decreasing creep

6-7. Denture materials should have high thermal conductivity for:
(a) Relishing hotness, taste   (b) Resist softening
(c) Dimensional stability   (d) Decreasing creep

6-8. Aesthetic requirements of denture materials:
(a) Transparency
(b) Ability to incorporate desired coloured pigments
(c) Stable hue, chroma and values
(d) All of the above

6-9. PMMA denture material (heat cure acrylic) has compressive strength in MPa:
(a) 16–18   (b) 75
(c) 380   (d) 2,450

6-10. PMMA denture material (heat cure acrylic) has modulus of elasticity in MPa:
(a) 16–17   (b) 75
(c) 380   (d) 2,450

6-11. PMMA heat cure acrylic denture base has surface hardness in KHN:
(a) 16–18   (b) 75
(c) 380   (d) 2,450

6-12. PMMA heat cure acrylic denture base has specific gravity:
(a) 0.945   (b) 1.19
(c) 4.51   (d) 10.5

6-13. Heat cure acrylic denture base monomer has specific gravity:
(a) 0.945   (b) 1.19
(c) 4.51   (d) 10.5

6-13a. Polymerisation volume shrinkage of methyl methaacrylate monomer:
(a) 7.0%   (b) 11.4%
(c) 21%   (d) 37%

6-14. Normal boiling temperature of methyl metha acrylate liquid in °C is:
(a) 48.3
(b) 100.8
(c) 152.5
(d) 779

6-15. PMMA (heat cure acrylic) satisfies the ideal requirements for denture material, with respect to:
(a) Mechanical
(b) Thermal
(c) Biological and aesthetics
(d) All of the above

6-16. The present commonly used non-metallic denture base material is:
(a) Vulcanite
(b) Bakelite
(c) Poly carbonates
(d) Poly methyl methacrylate

6-17. Initiator in heat cure acrylic DB material is:
(a) Heat
(b) Benzoyl peroxide
(c) Camphoroquinone
(d) Benzoin methyl ether

6-18. Activator in self cure acrylic DB material is:
(a) Visible light of $\lambda = 468$ nm
(b) Benzoyl peroxide
(c) Dimethyl para toluidine
(d) Benzoin methyl ether

6-19. Cross-linking agent in DB acrylic materials is:
(a) Glycol dimetha acrylate
(b) Benzoyl peroxide
(c) Dimethyl paratoluidine
(d) Benzoin methyl ether

6-20. Common denture fabrication technique is by:
(a) Light curing
(b) Heat curing-compression moulding
(c) Sintering
(d) Self curing fluid resin method

6-21. Three-mix-flasking technique of wax denture is done to get:
(a) Stronger denture
(b) Better aesthetics
(c) Plaster-free denture
(d) Recovery without fracture

6-22. Separating medium used at present is:
(a) Alginate sol.
(b) Tin foil
(c) Cellulose lacquers
(d) Soap solution

6-23. Separating medium contains dissolved alginate salt about:
(a) 85–88%
(b) 2–3%
(c) 7%
(d) 100%

6-24. Separating medium is mainly used for:
(a) Separation of denture from plaster
(b) Bonding acrylic teeth to denture
(c) Prevent diffusion of monomer into plaster
(d) Easy removal of denture from flask

6-25. Separating medium if applied on the exposed tooth surface:
(a) Prevents bonding of acrylic teeth
(b) Decreases strength of dentures
(c) Reduces surface hardness
(d) Causes discolouration

6-26. Polymer/powder ratio of about 2.5:1 by volume or 3:1 by weight, is mixed with monomer liquid to form a dough to:
(a) Reduce polymerisation shrinkage
(b) Facilitate packing
(c) Get dimensional accuracy
(d) All of the above

6-27. Dough time becomes shorter if:
(a) Degree of polymerisation is lower
(b) More plasticizer
(c) Higher temperature
(d) All of the above

6-28. Bench curing for half an hour eliminates:
(a) Irregular shrinkage microporosity
(b) Boiling monomer porosity
(c) Air inclusion porosity
(d) Crazing of denture

6-29. **Exothermic polymerisation heat produced by MMA (in cal/gm mol) is:**
(a) 547
(b) 3,900
(c) 12,500
(d) 80

6-30. **Heat curing of acrylic denture is done at 70°C for 8 hrs to avoid:**
(a) Boiling monomer porosity
(b) Micro porosity
(c) Subsurface porosity
(d) Air inclusions

6-31. **Lack of pressure during curing causes:**
(a) Large regular voids
(b) Large irregular voids, and opacity
(c) Sub-surface porosity
(d) All of the above

6-32. **Fast curing technique is used to:**
(a) Improve the mechanical properties
(b) Reduce chance of crazing
(c) Good colour stability
(d) Save curing time

6-33. **Termination of polymerisation takes place by:**
(a) Hydrogen ion transfer
(b) Collision of growing polymer, with free radicals
(c) Collision with another growing chain
(d) Any one

6-34. **Bench (or slow) cooling is done to:**
(a) Improve the mechanical properties
(b) Reduce chance of crazing
(c) Get good colour stability
(d) Plaster-free denture

6-35. **Acrylic dentures are finally polished by:**
(a) Roughe
(b) Diamond paste
(c) Fine 180 grit sand or emery papers
(d) French-chalk

6-36. **Well-polished denture has:**
(a) Better aesthetics
(b) Less debris accumulation
(c) Least irritation to opposing soft tissues
(d) All of the above

6-37. **Acrylic dentures are kept in cold water whenever not used to:**
  (a) Avoid crazing
  (b) Prevent attack from insects
  (c) Preserve aesthetics
  (d) Not required

6-38. **Self curing acrylic denture has advantages:**
  (a) Shorter processing time
  (b) Better fit
  (c) Less porosities
  (d) All of the above

6-39. **Self cured denture has disadvantages:**
  (a) Inferior mechanical properties
  (b) Poor colour stability (yellowing)
  (c) Lower wear resistance
  (d) All of the above

6-40. **Micro-wave curing has the advantages:**
  (a) Homogeneous curing
  (b) Shorter processing time
  (c) Less internal porosities
  (d) All of the above

6-41. **Fluid resin (pour and cure) technique has advantages:**
  (a) Simpler and quicker technique
  (b) Less damage to artificial teeth
  (c) Minimal finishing and polishing
  (d) All of the above

6-42. **Fluid resin (pour and cure) technique has disadvantage:**
  (a) Poor mechanical and aesthetic properties
  (b) Poor bonding of teeth
  (c) Shifting of teeth and decrease of vertical dimensions
  (d) All of the above

6-43. **Visible light cured denture base material, supplied as sheet or rope forms in light-proof pouches, contain:**
  (a) Camphoroquinone
  (b) Cross-linking agent UDMA
  (c) NN-di-methyl paratoluidine
  (d) All of the above

6-44. PMMA denture resins are strengthened by:
  (a) Carbon or E-glass fibres
  (b) Colloidal silica
  (c) Silver-copper eutectic alloy spherical particles
  (d) Diatomaceous earth

6-45. Processing stresses inducing internal strains or crazing are produced by:
  (a) Repeated drying and wetting
  (b) Porcelain teeth in acrylic dentures
  (c) Rapid cooling after curing
  (d) All of the above

6-46. Creep of acrylic denture is lower when:
  (a) Temperature is higher
  (b) Cross-linking is more
  (c) Degree of polymerisation is less
  (d) Plasticizers are more

6-47. Denture hard-liners are used for:
  (a) Corrections for miss-fitting
  (b) Absorption of large masticating energies causing pain
  (c) Enhancing blood circulation in affected tissue and assisting quicker curing
  (d) Strengthening of denture

6-48. Long time soft resilient denture liners are used for:
  (a) Correction to miss-fitting
  (b) Absorption of large masticating energies causing pain
  (c) Enhancing blood circulation in affected tissues and assisting quicker healing
  (d) Improving strength

6-49. The common resilient denture liner used is:
  (a) Polysilicones   (b) Reinforced PMMA resins
  (c) vulcanite   (d) Polysulphides

6-50. Short time-soft resilient tissue conditioners are used for:
  (a) Correction to miss-fitting
  (b) Absorption of large masticating energies causing pain
  (c) Enhancing blood circulation in affected tissues and assisting quicker curing
  (d) Improving strength

6-51. Addition polysilicone resilient liner has disadvantage:
(a) Poor bonding to acrylic denture
(b) Growth of *Candida albican*
(c) Difficulty for trimming and polishing
(d) All of the above

6-52. Fractured dentures are repaired by:
(a) Cold cure acrylic
(b) Addition polysilicone
(c) Epoxy resins
(d) Zinc poly carboxylate cement

6-53. Advantage of cold cure acrylic special trays:
(a) Simple method
(b) Less distortion of impression
(c) Less wastage of expensive impression materials
(d) All of the above

6-54. Which is NOT required for maxillofacial reconstructive materials?
(a) Soft skin-like texture
(b) High elastic modulus
(c) Stability of colour shades
(d) Ability to incorporate matching colours

6-55. Which is NOT used for maxillofacial reconstruction?
(a) Polysilicone
(b) Plasticized PMMA
(c) Composite restorative VLC resins
(d) Synthetic rubbers

6-56. Disadvantage of acrylic artificial teeth:
(a) Aesthetics   (b) Wear resistance
(c) Bonding to acrylic denture   (d) Bio-compatibility

6-57. Disadvantage of porcelain artificial teeth:
(a) Aesthetics   (b) Wear resistance
(c) Bonding to acrylic denture   (d) Bio-compatibility

6-58. Advantages of porcelain artificial teeth:
(a) Abrasion of opposing natural teeth
(b) Excellent aesthetics
(c) Clicking sound
(d) Brittleness

6-59. Acrylic resins are NOT used for:
- (a) Tissue conditioning
- (b) Temporary crowns and bridges
- (c) Occlusal splints
- (d) Veneers

6-60. Denture cleansers used are:
- (a) Common dentifrices
- (b) Mild detergents
- (c) Vinegar
- (d) Any one

7. Biocompatible Aspects of Dental Materials

Biocompatibility is the property of materials to remain harmoniously with the living tissues. These should not react and produce any toxic or injurious effects on the biological functions. Some of the materials used in dentistry may undergo biological degradations such as corrosions in the oral environments and produces adverse effects. Biocompatibility is determined from the interaction between the foreign materials and the body-tissues (pulp, mucosa, etc.) from localized cytotoxicity such as systematic responses, allergenicity, hypersensitivity, estrogenecity, etc.

7-1. Biodynamic-interaction between material and tissues takes place through:
- (a) Neutral fluid
- (b) Interface film
- (c) Alkaline medium
- (d) Cementum

7.2. Which of the following tests is included in the primary-in vitro screening tests?
- (a) Cytotoxicity
- (b) Genotoxicity
- (c) Both of the above
- (d) None of the above

7-3. In cytotoxic evaluation test, dental materials in fresh or cured state are placed directly in contact with:
- (a) Tissue culture cells or on the membranes overlying the tissue culture cells
- (b) Shaved skin of the animal
- (c) Exposed pulp
- (d) Blood, saliva and tissue fluid

7-4. **Name the test which investigates genetic mutations, chromosomal structures, DNA changes or any other genetic changes caused by the test materials:**
(a) Cytotoxicity
(b) Genotoxicity
(c) Systemic toxicity
(d) Hypersensitivity

7-5. **Which of the following test is included in the secondary–animal *in vivo* screening tests?**
(a) Systemic toxicity
(b) Inhalation test
(c) Skin irritation/sensitization
(d) All of the above

7-6. **Which of the following test is conducted on sub-human primates dogs, pigs, etc. for clinical trials:**
(a) Primary *in vitro* screening
(b) Secondary–animal *in vivo* screening
(c) Preclinical usage screening
(d) All of the above

7-7. **Which of the following tests is included in the Preclinical usage screening test?**
(a) Pulp and dentin usage
(b) Pulp-capping pulpotomy usage
(c) Endodontic usage
(d) All of the above

7-8. **In which of the following preclinical usage screening test, materials are placed in class V cavities, using ZnOE as a control for testing in 7 days?**
(a) Pulp and dentin usage
(b) Pulp-capping pulpotomy usage
(c) Endodontic usage
(d) All of the above

7-9. **Beryllium dust reaching the alveoli of lungs, cause chronic inflammation known as:**
(a) Berylliosis
(b) Silicosis
(c) Swelling
(d) Carcinoma

7-10. **Which of the following metals is biocompatible?**
(a) Titanium
(b) Beryllium
(c) Nickel
(d) Ionic mercury

7-11. Which component in polyether causes allergic problems?

(a) Aromatic sulphonic acid   (b) Colloidal silica

(c) Tin octoate   (d) Chloroplatinic acid

8. Restorative Dental-Materials Cements

Intense research is going on in developing permanent restorative materials possessing all the biological, physical, mechanical, thermal and aesthetic properties of our tooth structure. Still it is not successful, even now, to find a single material for conservative or endodontic treatments. Depending on the clinical situations, many materials, to integrate all the desired requirements, complicated clinical procedures and sophisticated technologies are to be intelligently adapted with highest clinical skill to achieve almost desired results and patients' satisfaction, in replacing the missing part of the tooth or missing teeth. Hence conservative methods are used to save the teeth.

8-1. Conservative dentistry deals with:

(a) Restoration of missing teeth

(b) Restoration of coronal parts

(c) Treatments of pulpal and periapical pathologies

(d) Interception and treatments of malocclusions

8-2. Endodontia deals with:

(a) Restoration of missing teeth

(b) Restoration of coronal parts

(c) Treatments of pulpal and periapical pathologies

(d) Interception and treatments of malocclusions

8-3. Restorative materials should be neutral to protect the pulp from:

(a) Chemical insults   (b) Thermal insults

(c) Fracture   (d) None

8-4. Restorative materials should have high compressive strength to resist:

(a) Fracture   (b) Abrasion

(c) Deformations   (d) Elastic recoveries

8-5. **Restorative materials should have approximate surface hardness in KHN:**
(a) 65   (b) 110
(c) 340   (d) 820

8-6. **To minimise micro-leakage, restorative materials should have COTE in ppm/°C:**
(a) Zero   (b) 8.4
(c) 11.4   (d) 24.6

8-7. **Coefficient of thermal conduction of restorative materials should be:**
(a) Zero or < 0.0016 cg units   (b) > 0.0022 cg units
(c) 8.6 ppm/°C   (d) 11.4 ppm/°C

8-8. **Classification of restorative materials is done to select most suitable material for:**
(a) Luting   (b) Particular restoration
(c) Cement bases   (d) Any

8-9. **Classification of restorative materials is done according to their reactive ingradients:**
(a) Neutral—ZnOE cements
(b) Alkaline—$Ca(OH)_2$ cement
(c) Acidic-alumino-silicate cements, phosphoric acid cements
(d) Any

8-10. **$Ca(OH)_2$ and ZnOE are used for restorations:**
(a) Temporary   (b) Intermediate
(c) Permanant   (d) Any

8-11. **ZnOE type lll resin bonded EBA cements are used for restorations:**
(a) Temperory   (b) Intermediate
(c) Permanant   (d) Pit and fissure sealant

8-12. **Silver amalgam, DFG, HN, N, PBM alloys are used for restorations:**
(a) Temporary   (b) Intermediate
(c) Permanent   (d) Any

8-13. **Permanent cementations are done by:**
(a) $ZnPO_4$ (b) ZnPolyC
(c) GI type I   (d) Any one

8-14. Ca(OH)₂ and ZnOE are used for:
   (a) Pulp protection
   (b) Temporary filling or cementations
   (c) Low strength base
   (d) Any one

8-15. Cement bases should have:
   (a) Compressive strength < 103 MPa
   (b) Low conductivity
   (c) Film thickness < 25 microns
   (d) None of these

8-16. Permanent luting cements should have:
   (a) Strength >75 MPa, and pseudo plasticity
   (b) Low conductivity
   (c) Film thickness < 25 microns
   (d) All of these

8-17. Temporary filling materials should have:
   (a) Strength >75 MPa
   (b) High conductivity
   (c) Low strength <35 MPa
   (d) Low film thickness < 25 microns

8-18. Gutta-percha, chloropercha and ZnOE are used for:
   (a) Pit and fissure sealant
   (b) Root canal fillings
   (c) Cementations
   (d) Temporary crowns and bridges

8-19. Cavity liners are thin suspensions of:
   (a) Ca(OH)₂   (b) ZnOE
   (c) GIC lll   (d) Any one

8-20. Micro leakage is reduced by:
   (a) Cavity varnishes
   (b) Cavity liners
   (c) Cavity bases
   (d) None of these

8-21. Accelerator used in ZnOE cements is:
   (a) Olive oil   (b) White rosin
   (c) CaCl₂ or Zn acetate   (d) Zn stearates

8-22. Resin bonded ZnOE–Kalginol-cement has:
- (a) Copal-resin
- (b) Ortho ethoxy benzoic acid
- (c) Synthetic or MMA resins
- (d) Epoxy resins

8-23. ZnOE setting reaction is:
- (a) Auto catalytic
- (b) Acid base
- (c) Chelate
- (d) All of the above

8-24. ZnOE cement is:
- (a) Neutral and of low strength
- (b) Obtundent
- (c) Thermal insulator
- (d) All of these

8-25. Non eugenol cement contains:
- (a) Ortho ethoxy benzoic acid
- (b) Alumina
- (c) Hexyl vanillate
- (d) All of the above

8-26. $ZnPO_4$ luting cement powder particle size is about:
- (a) < 5 μm
- (b) < 25 μm
- (c) > 40 microns
- (d) 0.23 mm

8-27. $ZnPO_4$ cement powder is prepared after:
- (a) Fritting
- (b) Sintering at 1000–1400°C
- (c) Milling
- (d) Homogenizing

8-28. In presence of Zn and Al, setting reaction of ZnO + H_3PO_4 produces:
- (a) $ZnPO_4$
- (b) Hopeite matrix
- (c) Cohesive Zn-AL-PO_4 matrix
- (d) $Zn(OH)_2$

8-29. PH of $ZnPO_4$ cement initially 2 or 3 becomes almost neutral in:
- (a) One hour
- (b) One day
- (c) One week
- (d) One month

8-30. Standard powder/liquid ratio for $ZnPO_4$ luting cement is:
- (a) 1:1
- (b) 1.4:1
- (c) 2.8:1
- (d) 4.8:1

8-31. Standard powder/liquid ratio for $ZnPO_4$ cement base is:
- (a) 1:1
- (b) 1.4 :1
- (c) 2.4 :1
- (d) 4.8:1

8-32. Consistency of $ZnPO_4$ luting cement (when 0.5 ml of standard mix is placed under 125 gm load for 10 min) is the diameter of the mix:
(a) 20 mm
(b) 25–30 mm
(c) 30 mm
(d) 30–35 mm

8-33. Consistency of $ZnPO_4$, cement-base (when 0.5 ml of standard mix is placed under 125 gm load for 10 min) is the diameter of the mix:
(a) 20 mm
(b) 25–30 mm
(c) 30 mm
(d) 30–35 mm

8-34. Compressive strength of $ZnPO_4$ luting cement, in MPa should be:
(a) < 35
(b) >75 = 80–100
(c) >100.3 = 110–130
(d) 140–170

8-35. Compressive strength of $ZnPO_4$ base-cement in MPa is:
(a) < 35
(b) >75, = 80–100
(c) >100.3 = 110–130
(d) 140–170

8-36. Modulus of elasticity of $ZnPO_4$ luting cement in MPa is:
(a) 2,435
(b) Similar to dentin 14,000
(c) Similar to enamel 48,000
(d) 90,000

8-37. $ZnPO_4$ cement base has advantage of:
(a) Lower solubility
(b) Good thermal insulator
(c) Adequate strength
(d) All of the above

8-38. Modification of $ZnPO_4$ cement is
(a) Zn hydrophosphate, Zn-fluoride cement
(b) Germicidal-silver or copper cements
(c) Zn silico-phosphate
(d) All of the above

8-39. Small increments of $ZnPO_4$ cement powder are first added to a few drops of mixing liquid to:
(a) Reduce initial acidity and increase working time
(b) Shorten mixing time
(c) Adjust consistency
(d) Diffuse heat of exothermic reaction

8-40. **Large increments of $ZnPO_4$ cement powder are later added to the drops of liquid to:**
(a) Reduce initial acidity and increase working time
(b) Shorten mixing time
(c) Adjust consistency
(d) Diffuse heat of exothermic reaction

8-41. **$ZnPO_4$ cement powder and liquid are mixed covering large area to:**
(a) Reduce initial acidity and increase working time
(b) Diffuse heat of exothermic reaction
(c) Adjust consistency
(d) Shorten mixing time

8-42. **Metal crown to tooth, zinc phosphate cementation failure takes place:**
(a) Within enamel   (b) Within metal
(c) At enamel surface   (d) At metal-crown surface

8-43. **Silicate cement has become obsolate mainly due to:**
(a) Strength
(b) Aesthetics
(c) Prolonged acidity and irritant to pulp
(d) High solubility

8-44. **Silicate cement became initially popular due to:**
(a) Film thinness   (b) Anticariogenic property
(c) Acidity   (d) Solubility

8-45. **Zn-silicophosphates–synthetic porcelain was mainly used for:**
(a) Intermediate restorations
(b) Luting of ceramic crowns
(c) Die material
(d) Any

8-46. **Zinc poly carboxylate cement liquid is 30–50% aqueous solution of:**
(a) Itaconic acid   (b) Poly acrylic acid
(c) Tartaric acid   (d) Methyl metha acrylate

8-47. **Setting action of zinc poly carboxylate cement is through $COOH^+$ and:**
(a) Zn^{++} (b) Ca^{++} of enamel
(c) Ca^{++}, Mg^{++}, H^+ ions   (d) Al^{+++}

8-48. Bonding of zinc poly C cement to enamel is through COOH⁺ and:

(a) Zn^{++} (b) Ca^{++} chelation

(c) Ca^{++}, Mg^{++}, H^+ ions   (d) Al^{+++}

8-49. Bonding of zinc poly C cement to dentin is through COOH⁺ and:

(a) Zn^{++}

(b) Ca^{++} of enamel by chelating

(c) Ca^{++}, Mg^{++}, H^+ ions

(d) Al^{+++}

8-50. Initial pH 1.8–3.0 of zinc poly C cement becomes almost neutral in:

(a) One hour   (b) One day

(c) One week   (d) One month

8-51. Biocompatibility of zinc polycarboxylate cement is due to:

(a) Weak acid, pH rising rapidly

(b) Large sized PAA molecules

(c) Complexes formed blocking dentine tubules

(d) All of the above

8-52. Zn poly C cement is mild cement, kind to the pulp, since:

(a) Weak acid, pH rising rapidly

(b) Large sized PAA molecules

(c) Complexes formed blocking dentinal tubules

(d) All of the above

8-53. Zinc polycarboxylate tooth-metal cementation failure is at:

(a) Within enamel   (b) Within metal

(c) Enamel surface   (d) Metal-crown surface

8-54. Properties of Zn poly C cements:

(a) Biocompatible, chemically bonding with enamel and dentin but not to HN, N, PBM, alloys

(b) Mechanical properties slightly inferior to $ZnPO_4$ cement

(c) Thermal insulator, low COTE

(d) Opaque

8-55. Manipulation steps of Zn poly C cements:
(a) Measuring scoop and standard droppers are used
(b) P/L = 1.5 gm/ml or 2 drops/scoop—for cementation
(c) P/L = 2.3 gm/ml or one drop/scoop—for base
(d) Mix quickly first half, then other 2 halves by stropping folding or overlapping methods
(e) Apply on cementing crown surface before cobwebbing

8-56. Glass ionomer cement (prepared by fritting), powder has mainly:
(a) ZnO + MgO
(b) ZnO + Al_2O_3
(c) ZnO + SiO + Al_2O_3
(d) SiO + Al_2O_3 + Ca, Al, Na fluorides

8-57. Glass ionomer cement liquid is 45–50% aqueous solution of:
(a) Poly acrylic acid 45–50%
(b) Itaconic acid, maleic acid
(c) Tartaric acid
(d) All of the above

8-58. Type one, glass ionomer cement is used for:
(a) Restorations
(b) Luting
(c) Cavity liners and bases
(d) Pit and fissure sealing

8-59. Type two GIC is used for:
(a) Restorations
(b) Luting
(c) Cavity liners and bases
(d) Pit and fissure sealing

8-60. Type three GIC is used for:
(a) Restorations
(b) Luting
(c) Cavity liners, bases
(d) Pit and fissure sealing

8-61. Type four GIC is used for:
(a) Pit and fissure sealing
(b) Luting
(c) Cavity liners, bases
(d) Restorations

8-62. Type six GIC is used for:
(a) Restorations
(b) Core building
(c) Cavity liners, bases
(d) Pit and fissure sealing

8-63. Fuji-types 8 and 9—high viscosity GICs are used for:
(a) Restorations
(b) Atraumatic restorations-ART-gaediatric or paediatric materials
(c) Cavity liners, bases
(d) Luting

8-64. Setting action of GICs is through COOH$^+$ and:
(a) Zn^{++} (b) Ca^{++}
(c) Ca^{++}, Mg^{++}, H$^+$ ions   (d) Al^{+++}

8-65. Bonding of GIC with tooth enamel is through COOH$^+$ and:
(a) Zn^{++} (b) Ca^{++}
(c) Ca^{++}, Mg^{++}, H$^+$ ions   (d) Al^{+++}

8-66. Bonding of GIC with dentin is through COOH$^+$ and:
(a) Zn^{++} (b) Ca^{++}
(c) Ca^{++}, Mg^{++}, H$^+$ ions   (d) Al^{+++}

8-67. Special property of GIC is:
(a) Bio-compatibility   (b) Anti cariogenic
(c) Chemical bonding to tooth   (d) All of the above

8-68. Initial pH of 1.8–3.0, of GIC becomes almost neutral in:
(a) One hour   (b) One day
(c) One week   (d) One month

8-69. GIC is mild and kind to pulp, due to:
(a) Weak acid, pH rising rapidly
(b) Large sized PAA molecules
(c) Complexes formed block dentine tubules
(d) All of the above

8-70. Initial losely bound water, later binds tightly which?
(a) Increases solubility   (b) Increases strength
(c) Decreases strength   (d) Has no effect

8-71. Anticariogenic property of GIC is due to:
(a) Formation of less soluble fluoroapatite
(b) Inhibition of carbohydrate metabolism
(c) Inhibition of enzyme activity
(d) All of the above

8-72. GIC is used as bone substitute (cement) in maxillofacial surgeries hip-joint replacements, etc. due to:
(a) Suitable thermal and mechanical properties
(b) Osseo-integration through osteo-conductive ions
(c) Chemical adhesion to bones
(d) All of the above

8-73. GIC restorations have compression strengths in MPa:
(a) 6–7   (b) 70–100
(c) 140–150   (d) 8,000–9,000

8-74. GIC restorations have modulus of elasticity, in MPa:
(a) 2,450   (b) 8,000–9,000
(c) 18,000   (d) 41,400

8-75. Properties of GIC restorations:
(a) Biocompatible, chemically bonding with enamel and dentin but not to HN, N, PBM, alloys
(b) Mechanical properties higher than $ZnPO_4$
(c) Thermal insulator, low COTE- 13–16 ppm/°C
(d) Translucent-good aesthetics

8-76. Manipulation steps of GIC cements:
(a) Measuring scoop and standard droppers are used
(b) P/L = 1.25–1.5 gm/ml. Or 2 drops/scoop for cementation
(c) P/L = 3 gm/ml. one drop/scoop for restorations
(d) Mix quickly first half, then other 2 halves by stropping, folding or overlapping technique in minimum area, with agate/plastic spatula
(e) Use before cob-webbing
(f) Preshaped matrix bands are used to get proper shape, smooth surface and protect from moist environment (or apply varnish to prevent drying of surface during setting period)

8-77. Contraindications to use GIC in contact with ZnOE, since it:
(a) Prevents bonding to tooth
(b) Causes opacity
(c) Is a solvent to acrylics
(d) None of the above

8-78. Drawbacks of GIC:
(a) Slow setting
(b) Low shear strength
(c) Brittleness and inadequate strength
(d) All of the above

8-79. Metal-modified GIC of Dr Siemans—miracle mix, GIC powder is included with:
(a) Composite resins
(b) Spherical silver amalgam alloy
(c) Silver or gold powders
(d) Base-metal alloys

8-80. Metal-modified GIC of Dr Maclean's - Cermet (ceramics + metal), GIC powder is included with:
(a) Composite resins
(b) Silver amalgam alloy
(c) Silver or gold fine dust
(d) Base metal alloys

8-81. Drawback of metal modified GICs:
(a) Strength   (b) Poor aesthetics
(c) Both   (d) None of these

8-82. Resin-modified-GIC, powder is included with:
(a) Composite resins with photoinitiators
(b) Silver or gold dust
(c) Silver amalgam alloy
(d) Glycol dimethacrylate

8-83. Resin modified GIC, i.e., Compomer, Resinomer, Hybrid ionomers have:
(a) Anticariogenic propertion
(b) Chemically bonding to tooth
(c) Good aesthetics
(d) All of the above

8-84. Resin bonded tricure compomers dispensed as single paste sets by:
(a) Acid-base
(b) Chemically curing through benzoyl peroxide
(c) Light curing through camphoroquinone
(d) All of the above

8-85. Resin bonded tricure compomers have:
   (a) Chemically bonding to tooth
   (b) Adequate aesthetics
   (c) Dentist's command set property
   (d) All of the above

8-86. Tricure GIC is suitable for:
   (a) Core build up material
   (b) Cementation of ceramic crowns
   (c) Liners and fissure sealants
   (d) Any of these

8-87. Advantages of GIC liners:
   (a) Anticariogenic, biocompatibility
   (b) Direct bonding to tooth
   (c) Thermal insulator
   (d) All of the above

8-88. Sandwich technique refers to:
   (a) Silver amalgam with base
   (b) Composite with GICs
   (c) Double impression technique
   (d) Metal modified GIC

8-89. Barriers to the passage of irritants from cements are:
   (a) Restorations   (b) Pit-fissure sealants
   (c) Cement bases   (d) Cavity liners

8-90. Protection of pulp from-trauma, chemical, thermal and electrical insults is done by:
   (a) Cavity liners and bases   (b) Metallic restorations
   (c) Zinc phosphate cements   (d) Pit and fissure sealants

8-91. Requirements of cement bases:
   (a) Stimulate formation of secondary reparative dentin
   (b) Insulator, neutral or slightly alkaline
   (c) Strength, bonding to tooth
   (d) All of the above

8-92. Light cured Ca(OH)$_2$ cement—Dycal® contains:
   (a) Urethane dimethacrylate and camphoroquinone
   (b) Itaconic acid
   (c) Poly acrylic acid
   (d) Glycol salycilate

8-93. Ca (OH)$_2$ cement base is:
(a) Good conductor of heat
(b) Insulator, alkaline pH = 12
(c) Neutral, pH = 6–7
(d) Strong

8-94. Ca (OH)$_2$ low strength cement base is:
(a) Conductor of heat
(b) Anticariogenic
(c) Promoting growth of reparative dentin
(d) Chemically bonding to tooth

8-95. Gutta Percha (trans-isomer of poly isoprene) and Chloropercha thermoplastic cones/rods are used in dentistry for:
(a) Cement base
(b) Cavity lining
(c) Pit-fissure sealant
(d) Root canal filling/functional impressions

8-96. Approximate properties of common restoratives-cements:

Table 1.8.1					
Properties/ Materials	*CS MPa*	*TS MPa*	*Q orE, GPa*	*SH KHN. ppm/°C*	*COTE*
Ca(OH)$_2$	10–27	<1.5	0.4–1.2	Low	Low
ZnOE-l	30–40	0.3–6	2.2–5.4	—	—
Resin-ZnOE	45–55	4–5	2.5	—	—
ZnPO$_4$-luting	75–100,	5–5, 6.0	14–15	30–40,	—
ZnPO$_4$-base	100.3–170		22–24	40–50	
ZnPolyC	52–56	6–7	5 6	25 40	—
Zn-Si-PO$_4$—1	140	6.5	70	65	9–10
Zn-Si-PO$_4$—2	170	7.5	70	68	9–10
GIC-l	80–100	6–7	7–8	13–16	13–16
GIC-ll	190–250	1	8–9	25–40	11.6
Hybrid-composites	300–350	40–50	11–15	25–60	30–40
Ag-Amgm - High-Cu, single composition	One-hour 250–270	1-week- 65–70	4—60	100–110	22–28
Tooth enamel	330–380	10–11	40–70	340–345	11.4
Tooth dentin	300–350	50–53	14–18	65–70	8–6

Note: All materials, except silver amalgam, have very low thermal conductivities, e.g. Tooth enamel = 0.0022, dentin = 0.0016 cg units

9. Composite Restorative Resins

Excellent aesthetic properties of polymer resins, lead to the innovations of varities of visible light cured composite resins suitable for anterior or posterior restorations, pit and fissure sealants, etc., during later part of 20th century, by Dr Ray L Bowen (1962) and others by modifying acrylic resins.

The term composite resin refers to a three dimensional structure of at least two, or more, chemically different materials insoluble in each other, with a distinct interface separating the components.

9-1. Advantages of unfilled restorative acrylic resins used earlier:
(a) Aesthetics and simple method
(b) Strength
(c) High COTE.
(d) Polymerisation shrinkage

9-2. Disadvantages of unfilled restorative acrylic resins used earlier:
(a) Poor strength
(b) Pulpal irritations
(c) Large polymerisation shrinkage
(d) All of the above

9-3. Bulk-pack, pressure, or incremental bead techniques are used for:
(a) Poly ethers
(b) Zinc phosphate cementation
(c) Gutta percha
(d) Unfilled acrylic resin restorations

9-4. Common organic resin matrix used in Bowen's composite resins is:
(a) Triethelene glycol dimethacrylate
(b) Viscous bisphenol glycidyl dimethacrylate–with or without -OH group
(c) Blend of BisGMA and TEGDMA
(d) Blend of poly acrylic and itaconic acids

9-5. Composite resins have pyrolytic precipitated glass powder to:
(a) Bond with resin matrix
(b) Bond with tooth
(c) Improve strength
(d) Initiate setting

9-6. Inorganic pyrolytic precipitated glass fillers in composite resins:
(a) Decreases thermal expansion and setting shrinkage
(b) Improves aesthetics
(c) Improves strength
(d) All of the above

9-7. Filler percentage by weight in hybrid posterior all purpose composite resins:
(a) 20–30
(b) 35–65
(c) 75–80
(d) 85–92

9.8. Coupling agents in composite restorative resins:
(a) Titanates, zirconates
(b) Vinyal silane
(c) Gama metha acryloxy tri-methoxy silane
(d) Any one

9.9. Coupling agents in composite restorative resins:
(a) Increases strength
(b) Decreases COTE
(c) Acts as stress absorber
(d) All of these

9-10. Composite restorative resins contain camphoroquinone to:
(a) Bond with resin matrix
(b) Initiate setting of VLC
(c) Improve strength
(d) Chemical activation

9-11. Composite restoratives contain benzoin methyl ether to:
(a) Bond with resin matrix
(b) Initiate UV curing-setting
(c) Improve strength
(d) Bond with tooth

9-12. Chemically cured composite resins contain BHT (butylated hydroxyl toluene) to:
(a) Accelerate polymerisation
(b) Increase working time and shelf-life
(c) Improve strength
(d) Initiate setting

9-13. Chemically cured composite resins contain NN dimethyl-p-toludene to:
(a) Accelerate or activate polymerisation
(b) Increase working time and shelf-life
(c) Improve strength
(d) Initiate setting

9-14. Wave length of visible light used for curing of resins in "nm" is:
(a) 350   (b) 468
(c) 689.3   (d) 987

9-15. Filler particle size of microfilled composite resins, in microns is:
(a) 0.00046   (b) 0.04–0.06
(c) 0.4–1   (d) 8–12

9-16. Initiators for VLC composites is:
(a) Benzoil peroxide
(b) Benzoin methyl ether
(c) Camphoroquinone
(d) Visible light of wave length = 468 nm

9-17. Composite resin of highest compressive and tensile strength is:
(a) Micro filled
(b) Small particles
(c) Hybrid small particle
(d) Traditional large particle

9-18. Which composite resin has highest abrasion resistance?
(a) Microfilled   (b) Small particles
(c) Hybrid   (d) Traditional large particle

9-19. Which composite resin has best polishability?
(a) Microfilled   (b) Small particles
(c) Hybrid   (d) Traditional large particle

9-20. Which composite resin has highest resistance to deformations (i.e. modulus of elasticity)?
(a) Micro filled
(b) Small particles
(c) Hybrid
(d) Traditional large particle

9-21. Which composite resin has least mechanical properties?
(a) Microfilled
(b) Flowable hybrid
(c) Posterior-hybrid
(d) Traditional

9-22. Curing shrinkage % of composite restorative resins is about:
(a) Negligible
(b) 2–3
(c) 4–7
(d) 11–13

9-23. Composite restorative resins have COTE (in ppm/°C) about:
(a) 11–15
(b) 25–30
(c) 80–120
(d) 150–225

9-24. Hybrid, direct posterior dense composites have adequate:
(a) Compression strength
(b) Abrasive resistance, aesthetics
(c) Resistance to deformations
(d) All of the above

9-25. Indirect composite resins are used as:
(a) Core-build ups
(b) Posterior restorations
(c) Pre fabricated inlays, onlays
(d) Resin crowns

9-26. Flowable composite restorations are used for:
(a) Inaccessible class 1 or 2 restorations
(b) Pit and fissure sealants
(b) None of these
(d) Any one

9-27. Advantageous property of UV light (λ = 350 nm) cured composite restorative resins:
(a) Low depth of curing
(b) Decrease of intensity with time
(c) Need warming up time
(d) Command set property

9-28. Advantageous property of visible light light (λ = 468 nm) cured composite restorative resins:
(a) Higher depth of curing
(b) No health hazards
(c) Command set property
(d) All of the above

9-29. Curing time of VLC cured composite restoration is 20 secs when the tip of the light source is at 2 mm. What is the curing time when it is held at 2.0 cm distance?
(a) Same
(b) 40 sec
(c) 200 sec
(d) 30 min, 20 secs

9-30. Light source for curing composite resins is:
(a) LED
(b) Quartz tungsten halogen
(c) Plasma arc,or argon Lasers (λ = 490 nm)
(d) Any

9-31. Recent light source for curing composite resins is:
(a) LED
(b) Quartz tungsten halogen
(c) Plasma arc
(d) Argon lasers (λ = 490 nm)

9-32. Preventive resin restorations (for pit and fissures) are done by using:
(a) Microfilled or less loaded filler composites
(b) Hybrid composites
(c) Epoxy resins
(d) Unfilled acrylics

10. Bonding of Restorations

Many techniques and materials are used for mechanical and chemical bonding of varieties of restorative materials to tooth enamel and dentin for reducing marginal leakage and a longer life involving the principles of—wetting of surfaces, micromechanical interlocking, Chemical bonding and interpenetration forming hybrid zones.

10-1. The first bonding agent developed by Oskar Hagger (1940s) for both enamel and dentin bonding was:
(a) Gluteraldehyde
(b) Glycerophosphoric acid dimethacrylate
(c) 4-META
(d) Cyanoacrylates

10-2. Advantages of chemical adhesion of restorative materials to tooth structure are:
(a) Conservation of more natural tooth structure
(b) Optimum retention
(c) Prevention of microleakage
(d) All of the above

10-3. Acid etching technique was introduced to dentistry by:
(a) Bowen
(b) Michael Buonocore
(c) Dr Wilson
(d) Dr Kent

10-4. Acid etching of enamel is done with:
(a) Benzoyl peroxide   (b) 10% H_3PO_4
(c) 37% H_3PO_4 (d) HCl

10-5. Technique of etching simultaneously both dentin and enamel using 37% phosphoric acid is:
(a) Bond etch   (b) Acid etch
(c) Self etch   (d) Total etch

10-6. Optimum time for acid etching of enamel is about:
(a) 10 sec   (b) 20 sec
(c) 1.0 min   (d) 2.2 min

10-7. Acid etching of enamel produces shear bond strength with composite resin is about:
(a) 2–5 MPa   (b) 15–20 MPa
(c) 34 MPa   (d) 42 MPa

10-8. Acid etching produces a micro porosities (resin tags) on the enamel surface of about 6 µm in diameter and depth:
(a) 2–4 µm   (b) 10–20 µm
(c) 60–70 µm   (d) 1.6 mm

10-9. **Dentin etching is more technique sensitive than enamel etching because of:**
   (a) Complex structure-HAP crystal and Type I collagen
   (b) Dentinal fluid
   (c) Smear layer
   (d) All of the above

10-10. **Collagen network should be retained during dentin etching for the infiltration of:**
   (a) Primers   (b) Etchants
   (c) Water   (d) All of the above

10-11. **Which generations of dentin bonding agent is classified as self etch adhesives?**
   (a) 3rd and 4th
   (b) 4th and 5th
   (c) 5th and 6th
   (d) 6th and 7th

10-12. **Which generation of dentin bonding agent is classified as etch-and-bond?**
   (a) 3rd and 4th   (b) 4th and 5th
   (c) 5th and 6th   (d) 6th and 7th

10-13. **One-step or "All-in-one" adhesive is referred to which generation of bonding agent?**
   (a) 4th   (b) 5th
   (c) 6th   (d) 7th

10-14. **Which restorative material is NOT chemically bonding to tooth?**
   (a) Zn Poly C   (b) GIC
   (c) ZnOE   (d) Compomer

10-15. **Which restorative material is chemically bonding to tooth?**
   (a) ZnOE   (b) GIC
   (c) Zinc phosphate cement   (d) Composite resin

10-16. **Which restorative material is chemically bonding to tooth?**
   (a) Kalginol   (b) Dycal
   (c) Silver amalgam   (d) Compomer

11. Direct Filling Gold

Four nines (99.99% purity) gold restoration has perhaps longest history (about 2,500 BC) in dentistry. This is an ideal restorative if perfectly compacted. However, it has become obsolete due to impossibility to achieve perfectness in compaction, inadequate mechanical, thermal, aesthetic properties and also the availability of better recent materials and simple techniques.

Pure gold has FCC lattice, specific gravity = 19.3, MP = 1063°C. high conductivity, ductility, malleability and cold-welding properties.

Classifications according to manufacturing and dispensing methods.

1. Hammered-sheets—foils (of no.s 3,4,5, etc.), laminated, Preformed (ropes, cylinders,—), carbonized (corrugated), cohessive-noncohessive, platinised (mat-foil).
2. Electrolytic precipitate—mat (crystalline, spongy-sintered strips) mat-foil, electralloy (with a trace of calcium).
3. Chemically precipitated-granulated—golden EZ (encapsulated-powder in wax), stop-foil (sintered in between foils).

11-1. Who recently introduced pure gold restorations to dentistry?
   (a) Pierre Fauchard-1750   (b) Pfaff-1760
   (c) GV Black-1895   (d) Taggart-1897

11-2. Advantageous properties of DFG:
   (a) Mechanical strength properties
   (b) Thermal properties
   (c) High density
   (d) Excellent biocompatibility, cold weldability

11-3. Disadvantageous properties of DFG:
   (a) Cold weldability
   (b) Strength, thermal, aesthetics
   (c) Biological
   (d) Ductility, malleabilities

11-4. Verities of fibrous gold foil is initially obtained from:
   (a) Electrolytic ppt   (b) Sintering
   (c) Hammering   (d) Chemical ppt

11-5. Verities of spongy-mat-gold are initially obtained from:
(a) Electrolytic ppt   (b) Tempering
(c) Hammering   (d) Chemical ppt

11-6. Granulated powder—EZ-DFG is initially obtained from:
(a) Electrolytic ppt   (b) Tempering
(c) Hammering   (d) Chemical ppt

11-7. Surface contamination of DFG is prevented by:
(a) Sintering
(b) Desorption heat treatment
(c) Carbonizing
(d) Treating with NH_3 gas

11-8. Surface contaminations of DFG are removed by:
(a) Sintering   (b) Desorption heat treatment
(c) Carbonizing   (d) Treating with NH_3 gas

11-9. Indications to DFG restorations:
(a) Inlays and onlays
(b) Thick crowns
(c) Pit and fissure sealing
(d) Small fillings in non-stress bearing areas

11-10. Cement base is needed for DFG restoration, as it has:
(a) Low strength
(b) Cold weldability
(c) High thermal conductivity
(d) Surface impurities

11-11. Cavity varnish is applied before DFG restoration, since DFG has:
(a) Low strength
(b) High thermal conductivity
(c) No chemical bonding with tooth
(d) surface impurities

11-12. Noncohesive DFG is made cohesive by:
(a) Annealing at half of its MP in °K
(b) Homogenizing at 1000°C
(c) Sintering at 779°C
(d) Desorption heat treatment at about 400°C

11-13. Compaction of DFG is done using hand or mechanical pneumatic condensers by:
(a) Wedging
(b) Stepping
(c) Without bridging
(d) All including

11-14. With highest clinical skill, it is possible to achieve maximum DFG restoration density in gm/cc is only:
(a) 4–5
(b) 8.8383
(c) 16.0
(d) 19.3

11-15. With highest clinical skill, it is possible to achieve maximum flexure strength of DFG restoration (in MPa) is:
(a) 138
(b) 270
(c) 430
(d) 800

11-16. With highest clinical skill, it is possible to achieve maximum surface hardness of DFG restoration (in KHN) is:
(a) 24
(b) 69
(c) 110
(d) 800

Note: With highest clinical skill, it is not possible to eliminate voids, to get adequate mechanical properties and abrasive resistances. DFG restoration is an ideal one (gold standard), if performed perfectly. Since this is not possible, marginal leakage, debonding from cavity walls, failures, etc., result in worst restorations. Hence its use is very limited only to a few cases of nonstress-acting areas. At present it is very rarely used since many better aesthetic, stronger, more suitable materials can be used in a simpler manner, without causing fatigue to dentists.

12. Silver Amalgam Restorative Materials

GV Black's first formulation (in 1896) of Ag-Tin-Cu alloy and its later modifications reined the area of posterior teeth direct filling restorations during the last century even against the odds of toxicity and health hazards of mercury. However, the present researches on posterior-hybrid composite resins, and CAD-CAM technologies, etc., have almost lead to its banning!

12-1. Dental amalgam is an alloy of mercury with:
(a) Silver
(b) Tin, copper
(c) Silver, tin, copper
(d) Zinc, copper

12-2. Dental amalgam was introduced by:
(a) Dr Wilson
(b) Pierre Fauchard
(c) GV Black
(d) Bowen

12-3. The best variety of alloy used in silver amalgam is:
(a) Low copper lathe cut
(b) silver copper eutectic alloy
(c) High copper-admix alloy
(d) High copper-single composition alloy

12-4. Percentage of silver in low copper amalgam alloy is:
(a) 6 to 12
(b) 26–28
(c) 45–50
(d) 67–69

12-5. Silver in dental amalgam increases:
(a) Setting expansion
(b) Strength
(c) delayed expansion
(d) Creep

12-6. Melting temperature of silver is:
(a) 232°C
(b) 420°C
(c) 961°C
(d) 1083°C

12-7. Ordered gamma phase is formed from disordered beta phase by:
(a) Precipitation
(b) Homogenisation
(c) Peritectic transformation
(d) Eutectic change

12-8. Strongest phase in low-copper silver amalgam is:
(a) Beta phase
(b) Gama
(c) Gama-1
(d) Gama-2

12-9. Weakest phase in low-copper silver amalgam is:
(a) Beta
(b) Gama
(c) Gama-1
(d) Gama-2

12-10. Gama-2 (tin-mercury) phase of silver amalgam has lowest:
(a) Strength
(b) Corrosion resistance
(c) Dimensional stability
(d) All of the above

12-11. Intermeshing of Gama-1 by η-Cu_6Sn_5 phase is formed in:
(a) Low copper lathe-cut
(b) Disperse
(c) Spherical
(d) High copper single composition amalgam

12-12. Amalgam phase responsible for highest strength and lowest creep is formed by:
(a) Intermeshing of η-Cu_6Sn_5 phase with Gama-1
(b) Gama
(c) Gama-1
(d) Gama-2

12-13. Compressive strength of amalgam is high when:
(a) Hg/alloy is least
(b) Condensation force is high
(c) Optimum trituration
(d) All of the above

12-14. Maximum one-hour compressive strength of high copper amalgams in MPa is:
(a) 110
(b) 140
(c) 270
(d) 430

12-15. Max. tensile strength of silver amalgam restoration in MPa is about:
(a) 68
(b) 162
(c) 930
(d) 1760

12-16. Factor which increases setting expansion of silver amalgam:
(a) High Hg/alloy ratio
(b) Prolonged trituration
(c) Lower condensation force
(d) All of the above

12-17. Delayed expansion in Zn containing silver amalgam is due to:
(a) Low Hg/alloy ratio
(b) Prolonged trituration
(c) High condensation force
(d) Trapping of moisture

12-18. Creep of silver amalgam is lowest when:
(a) Hg/alloy is least
(b) Condensation force is high
(c) Optimum trituration
(d) All of the above

12-19. Criteria for selection of amalgam alloys:
(a) High 1 hour and max. strengths
(b) Low corrosion resistance
(c) Large setting expansion
(d) Large creep

12-20. Hg/alloy ratio by weight for high copper single composition alloy is about:
(a) 45%   (b) 54%
(c) 64%   (d) 72%

12-21. Increasing dryness restoration technique involves:
(a) Hg/alloy ratio > 50% by weight
(b) Squeezing of excess of Hg
(c) Removal of more Hg during condensation of every increment
(d) All of the above

12-22. Eame's technique involves:
(a) Hg/alloy ratio 1:1, by weight
(b) No squeezing of mix
(c) No removal of excess Hg during condensation
(d) All of the above

12-23. Trituration is required (as silver amalgam alloy particles are not wetted by Hg), due to:
(a) Large ST of Hg-465 dynes/cm
(b) Large angle of contact-135°
(c) Oxide layer on the alloy surface
(d) All of the above

12-24. Hg and alloys are dispensed by:
(a) Equal weights
(b) Measuring weight and volumes
(c) Using volume dispensers (1:1.5 ratio)
(d) None

12-25. **Hand-trituration time is about:**
(a) 25–30 sec
(b) 45–60 sec
(c) 3 min 15 sec
(d) 20 min

12-26. **Mechanical trituration time by using amalgamator is:**
(a) 25–30 sec
(b) 45–60 sec
(c) 3 min 15 sec
(d) 20 min

12-27. **Mechanical or hand mulling is done to:**
(a) Homogenise the mix
(b) Remove the excess of mercury
(c) Reduce condensation force
(d) Increase expansion

12-28. **Working time for triturated amalgam is about:**
(a) 45–60 sec
(b) 3 min15 sec
(c) 20 min
(d) 1 hr

12-29. **Amalgam cry-metallic scratching sound indicates:**
(a) Final setting of amalgam
(b) To initiate carving
(c) To stop carving
(d) None

12-30. **Clinically setting time of silver amalgam is:**
(a) 20 min
(b) one hour
(c) 8 hours
(d) 24 hours

12-31. **Amalgam condensation is done by a force about:**
(a) Negligible
(b) 1.6 kg
(c) 3.6 kg
(d) Max. the patient can withstand

12-32. **Purpose of condensation is to achieve:**
(a) Maximum density and strength
(b) Good adaptation to cavity walls
(c) Minimum dimensional change and creep
(d) All of the above

12-33. **The waste dental amalgam, alloy mercury miximum in clinics and laboratories should be stored in:**
(a) Sodium thio-sulphate solutions
(b) Amber colored bottle
(c) 50% hydrochloric acid
(d) Methyl methacrylate liquid

12-34. Carving, polishing and burnishing are required for:
(a) Aesthetics
(b) Minimise debris collection
(c) Lower corrosion resistance
(d) None of these

12-35. Which amalgam phase has least corrosion resistance?
(a) η-Cu_3Sn (b) Gama
(c) Gama-1   (d) Gama-2

12-36. To minimise (galvanic) corrosion of amalgam restorations:
(a) Avoid contact of dissimilar alloys
(b) Use low copper alloys
(c) Use high Hg/alloy ratio
(d) Leave the surface unfinished

12-37. Micromarginal-leakage in amalgam restorations is due to:
(a) Large difference in COTE wrt teeth
(b) Poor adaptation and bonding
(c) Marginal breakdowns
(d) All of the above

12-38. Micro-marginal-leakage in amalgam restorations can be reduced by:
(a) Using cavity varnishes
(b) Good adaptation
(c) Using high copper single composition alloy
(d) All these methods

12-39. Mercuroscopic expansion causes:
(a) Squeezing of mercury from margins
(b) Ditching of restorations
(c) Increases in tensile strength
(d) Increases in surface hardness

12-40. Amalgam bond contains mainly:
(a) Vinyl silane
(b) Polyalkenoates
(c) Ferric oxalate
(d) 4-META—methacryloxyethyl trimellitate anhydride

12-41. Advantages of spherical alloys amalgam:
(a) Lower Hg/alloy ratio—higher strength
(b) Lower condensation force
(c) Better surface finish
(d) All of the above

12-42. Disadvantage of spherical alloys amalgam:
(a) Too plastic mix-difficult to condense
(b) Higher strength
(c) Lower creep
(d) Lower mercuroscopic expansion

12-43. Disadvantage of amalgam restorations:
(a) Poor aesthetics
(b) No chemical bonding with teeth
(c) Mercury health hazards
(d) All of the above

12-44. Disadvantage of amalgam restorations:
(a) Poor bonding to teeth
(b) Require thermal insulating base
(c) Dimensional changes and microleakage
(d) All of the above

12-45. The gallium metal has the following property:
(a) Melting temp. 29.8°C
(b) Becomes liquid at room temperature on alloying with indium and tin
(c) Form gallium intermetallic phases with Cu, Ag, Pd and Sn.
(d) All of the above

12-46. Disadvantages of gallium alloys:
(a) Less mercury health hazards
(b) Too thin plastic mix and difficult to condense
(c) Good mechanical properties
(d) None

12-47. Advantage of indium containing silver alloy amalgam:
(a) High one hour strength (430 MPa)
(b) Low creep 0.06 to 0.1%
(c) Less mercury health hazard
(d) All of the above

12-48. Copper amalgam is supplied as pellets:
(a) When heated gives out mercury for trituration
(b) Large mercury content cause health hazards
(c) Shows poor corrosion resistance and mechanical properties
(d) All of the above

12-49. Symptom of mercury toxicity is:
(a) Fatigue and headaches
(b) Tingling sensation of extremities of the body
(c) Renal disorders
(d) All of the above

12-50. Thresh hold level (TLV) values prescribed by Occupational Safety Health Administration (OSHA) and ADA in atmosphere:
(a) 50 mg/m^3
(b) 3 mg/litre
(c) 7 mg/litre
(d) 4 mg/kg weight of person

12-51. Thresh hold level (TLV) values prescribed by occupational safety health administration (OSHA) and ADA in blood:
(a) 50 mg/m^3
(b) 3 microgm/ml
(c) 7 mg/litre
(d) 4 mg/kg weight of person

12-52. Thresh hold level values (TLV) prescribed by occupational safety health administration (OSHA) and ADA in Urine:
(a) 50 mg/m^3
(b) 3 mg/litre
(c) 7 mg/litre
(d) 4 mg/kg weight of person

12-53. The best alternative for silver amalgam restoration is:
(a) Hybrid composite resin
(b) Glass ionomer cement
(c) Dental ceramics
(d) Direct filling gold

13. Dental Ceramics

Search for restorative materials of adequate mechanical properties and excellent aesthetic qualities lead to the applications of ceramics, as metal bonded ceramics, all-ceramics verities, recent chair-side computer aided designing and machining (CAD CAM.), copy milling technologies, etc., in dentistry. Ceramics are non-metallic, inorganic, hard, high fusing, brittle materials of simple compounds of oxygen with one or more metallic or semi-metallic materials (like Si, Al, Ca, Li, Na, K, Mg, P, Ti, Zr, etc.). Diamond is the hardest (>10,000 KHN) and very high fusion temperature (>3,700°C) ceramic. In silicate glass, the silica atoms are bound to four oxygen atoms which link at random, other tetrahedral SiO_4, forming polymeric type $(SiO_2)_n$ structures, each oxygen atom linking with two silica atoms. Nonoxide ceramics such as nitrides of Al, B, Si, Ti, borides (Ti, Zr), carbides (Ti, B, Si, W—hard abrasives), zinc selinides, sialons, (Si_3N_4 with Al_2O_3, etc.) are not used commonly in dentistry due to their higher opacities, fusion temperatures, etc.

The glass formers are-silica, Al_2O_3, MgO, ZrO_2, etc., SiO^{4+} has tetrahedral structure.

The Glass-interrupters, or devitrifies are—metallic ions of K^+, Na^+, Al^{+++}, Ca^{++}, etc.

The four basic structural verities of ceramics are:
- Amorphous silicate ceramics (SiO_2, with small amounts of Al_2O_3, MgO, ZrO_2 etc.)
- Crystalline oxide ceramics with crystalline phases of Al_2O_3, MgO, ThO_2, ZrO_2 (MgO + Al_2O_3, $3Al_2O_3$ + $2SiO_2$, Al_2O_3 + TiO_2 used as refractory materials in Ti-alloy casting).
- Partially crystallised–stabilised ceramics—dicor, glass infiltrated ceramics, etc.
- Non-oxide ceramics-borides, carbides, silicides, nitrides, selenides, etc., which are rarely used in dentistry.

Various classifications are, according to:
- Compositions—feldspathic, leucite-based, lithia-based, aluminous, containing alumina, silica, zirconia.

- Processing technique—sintering in air, diffusible gases, or vacuum. Partial sintering and glass infiltration, hot pressing and slip casting, CAD-CAM, copy milling, etc.
- Placement verities—core, opaque, body (dentin), gingival-neck, cervical, enamel, colour-frits or pigments, glazes—porcelains.
- Fusion temperatures—high fusing >1300°C, medium 1100—1300°C, low-850° 1100°C, ultra-low < 850°C.

13-1. Ceramics have atomic bonding through:
  (a) Hydrogen   (b) Oxygen
  (c) Free electrons   (d) Halides

13-2. Dental ceramics have:
  (a) No ductility but brittleness
  (b) High conductivity
  (c) Large COTE
  (d) Low surface hardness

13-3. Dental ceramics have:
  (a) High ductility, elasticity   (b) Low conductivity
  (c) Large COTE   (d) Low surface hardness

13-4. Dental ceramics have:
  (a) High ductility, elasticity   (b) Large conductivity
  (c) Low COTE   (d) Low surface hardness

13-5. Dental ceramics have:
  (a) High ductility, elasticity   (b) Low conductivity
  (c) Large COTE   (d) All of the above

13-6. The impact strength of yitria stabilized zirconia or ceria stabilized alumina-zirconia in MPa-m$^{1/2}$ is:
  (a) 0.75   (b) 0.7–1.3
  (c) 3–1   (d) 8

13-7. All the properties of ceramics are due to:
  (a) Sintering   (b) Glass infiltration
  (c) Glazing   (d) Absence of free-electrons.

13-8. Glass-former—feldspar mineral ores refer to alumina silicates of:
  (a) Potash   (b) Soda
  (c) Lime   (d) Any one

13-9. Glass modifiers (interrupters) K^+, Na^+, Ca^{++} ions cause divitrification and decrease:
- (a) Fusion and glass-transition temperatures
- (b) hardness
- (c) Slip-resistance
- (d) All of the above

13-10. The binder-kaolin is a hydrated:
- (a) Alumino-silicate
- (b) Leucite
- (c) Feldspar
- (d) Metallic oxides

13-11. Feldspathic glazed porcelain has transverse strength in MPa:
- (a) 25
- (b) 140
- (c) 460
- (d) 70,000

13-12. Feldspathic porcelain has tensile strength in MPa:
- (a) 110
- (b) 343
- (c) 460
- (d) 2500

13-13. Ceramics have approximate surface hardness in KHN:
- (a) 22
- (b) 111
- (c) 460
- (d) 820

13-14. Feldspathic porcelain has COTE in ppm/°K:
- (a) 9–12
- (b) 11.4
- (c) 45–54
- (d) 81–120

13-15. Incongruent melting of feldspathic porcelain produce:
- (a) Castable glass
- (b) Leucite crystals
- (c) High viscous fluid
- (d) Incerams.

13–16. Leucite porcelain has COTE in ppm/°K:
- (a) 9–12
- (b) 11.4
- (c) 20–25
- (d) 81–120

13-17. During solidification of ceramics, large number microcracks are formed, since it is:
- (a) Transparent
- (b) Having low COTEs
- (c) Poor conductor of heat
- (d) Very brittle

13-18. Toughening of ceramics is done by:
- (a) Interruption of crack propagation
- (b) Introduction of residual surface compressive stresses
- (c) Avoiding sharp corners and wrinkles in design
- (d) All of the above

13-19. Dispersion toughening of ceramics is done by introducing:
(a) Hard alumina or luecite crystals
(b) Kaolin
(c) Partially stabilised zirconia
(d) Immersing soda verity ceramic in KNO_3 solution

13-20. Ion-exchange or chemical toughening is done by introducing:
(a) Hard alumina or luecite crystals
(b) Kaolin
(c) Partially stabilised zirconia
(d) Immersing soda verity ceramic in KNO_3 solution

13-21. Transformation toughening of ceramics is done by:
(a) Hard alumina or luecite crystals
(b) Kaolin
(c) Partially stabilised zirconia
(d) Immersing soda verity ceramic in KNO_3

13-22. Toughening by thermal bonding is done by:
(a) Mismatching COTE of adjacent layers
(b) Kaolin
(c) Partially stabilised zirconia
(d) Immersing soda verity ceramic in KNO_3

13-23. Condensation of porcelain slurry on adapted platinum foil is done by:
(a) Spatulation
(b) Brush technique
(c) Mechanical/ultrasonic, vibration methods
(d) All of the above

13-24. Careful condensation of porcelain slurry on adapted platinum foil is done for:
(a) Minimising firing volume shrinkage
(b) Avoiding glazing
(c) Resisting crack-propagation
(d) Lowering fusion temperature

13-25. Vacuum firing of ceramics and cooling under pressure:
(a) Lowers fusion temperature
(b) Minimises firing volume shrinkage

(c) Avoids glazing

(d) Increases opacity

13-26. Firing is stopped at the low bisque stage, for:

(a) Casting glasses

(b) Porcelain jacket crowns

(c) Porcelain fused to metals

(d) Inceram technique

13-27. High bisque stage firing is done for fabrications of:

(a) Cast glasses

(b) Porcelain jacket crowns

(c) Porcelain fused to metals

(d) All of the above

13-28. Prolonged firing after high bisque stage causes:

(a) Air inclusion voids

(b) Rough surfaces

(c) Volume contractions

(d) Pyro-plastic flow

13-29. Volume shrinkage on firing is compensated by:

(a) Adding extra slurry and re-firing

(b) Preparing pattern, over sized by 13–14% linear

(c) Any one

(d) None of these

13-30. Voids in porcelain firing are minimised by:

(a) Vacuum firing

(b) Cooling under pressure

(c) Firing under diffusible gasses

(d) All of the above

13-31. Finishing of porcelain articles is done by:

(a) Glazing

(b) Electropolishing

(c) Using zirconium slurry

(d) Fine emery paper

13-32. Glazed porcelain has:

(a) Higher COTE

(b) Increased refractive index

(c) Lower transverse strength

(d) Higher flexure strength-140 MPa

13-33. Ceramic viscous liquid does not wet and bond with metals easily since:
   (a) Ceramic liquids have large surface tension, 365 dynes/cm at 1000°C and angle of contact = 138°
   (b) Different COTEs
   (c) Metals have oxide layer
   (d) Metals have higher fusion temperatures

13-34. Metal-ceramic bonding is achieved by:
   (a) Mechanical-rough surface interlocking
   (b) Chemical-through SnO
   (c) Thermal-COTE-mismatching
   (d) All of the above

13-35. Compared to ceramics, metals used in metal-ceramics, should have fusion temperature:
   (a) Lower by 100°C   (b) Higher by 100°C
   (c) Slightly mismatching   (d) Equal

13-36. Compared to ceramics, metals used in metal-ceramics, should have COTE:
   (a) Lower by 12 ppm/°C   (b) Higher by 12 ppm/°C
   (c) Slightly mismatching   (d) Equal

13-37. Fusion temperature of metal-ceramics alloys can be raised by addition of:
   (a) Pt and Pd   (b) Ag or Cu eutectic compositions.
   (c) Gold   (d) Zinc

13-38. COTE of metal-ceramics alloys can be lowered by adding:
   (a) Pt or Pd   (b) Ag or Cu eutectic compositions
   (c) Gold   (d) Zinc

13-39. COTE of ceramics of metal-ceramics can be raised by:
   (a) Leucite   (b) devitrifies
   (c) Any of these   (d) None of these

13-40. Silver and coppers are contraindicated for metal-ceramic alloys since these:
   (a) Decrease fusion temp
   (b) Cause greening (discoloration)
   (c) Increase COTE
   (d) Change densities

13-41. PBM alloys are preferred for metal-ceramics since they have suitable:
(a) Biocompatibility and rigidity
(b) Higher fusion temperatures
(c) Chemical and thermal bondings
(d) All of the above

13-42. Causes for metal ceramics bond failures:
(a) Low strengths and porosities in ceramics
(b) Too thick, weaker oxide layer
(c) Inadequate thickness of oxide layer
(d) Any

13-43. Advantages of metal ceramics are:
(a) Higher strength, durability, fracture resistance
(b) Complicated fabrication technique
(c) Non-vital appearance
(d) All of the above

13-44. Disadvantages of metal ceramics are:
(a) Poorer aesthetics (at cervical regions)
(b) Flexure failure
(c) More removal of healthy tooths material
(d) All of the above

13-45. Modifications of metal ceramic techniques:
(a) Using swagged gold-foil
(b) Electrodeposition of gold and tin
(c) Bonded platinum foil
(d) All of the above

13-46. Ceramming of cast DICOR glass articles is done mainly for:
(a) Chameleon effect   (b) Glazing
(c) Decreasing tensile strength (d) Surface hardening

13-47. Injection moulding and hot-pressable, all glass articles have:
(a) Higher flexure strength and aesthetics
(b) Lower COTE
(c) Twice the tensile and shear strengths
(d) Resistance to discolouration

13-48. Alumina-core ceramics contain alumina core material:
(a) 27%
(b) 40–50%
(c) 90%
(d) 100%

13-49. Glass infiltration core of inceram is fired up to the stage:
(a) Low bisque
(b) Medium bisque
(c) High bisque
(d) Complete fusion

13-50. Which is NOT glass infiltrated inceram core?
(a) Al_2O_3 core
(b) Spinnel-MgO.Al_2O_3
(c) Zirconia
(d) Dicor glass

13-51. Which has highest (700 MPa) flexure strength?
(a) ICA—Al_2O_3 core
(b) ICS—Spinnel-MgO.Al_2O_3,core
(c) ICZ—Zirconia, Al_2O_3 = 70% + ZrO = 30% core
(d) Feldspathic ceramic

13-52. Advantages of CAD-CAM techniques:
(a) Selection of defect less toughest material
(b) Short time chair-side procedure
(c) Simpler laboratory procedures
(d) All of the above

13-53. Etchant used for ceramics to improve bonding is:
(a) HCl
(b) HF
(c) H_2SO_4
(d) H_3PO_4

13-54. Cementation of ceramic restorations is done, at present by:
(a) Zinc phosphate
(b) Silicate
(c) Zinc polycarboxylate
(d) Tri-cure compomer

13-55. Advantages of artificial ceramic teeth:
(a) Aesthetics
(b) Brittleness
(c) Impact strength
(d) Clicking sound

13-56. Disadvantages of artificial ceramic teeth:
(a) Abrasion of opposing tooth
(b) Brittleness, clicking sound
(c) No chemical boding with acrylics
(d) All of the above

13-57. Properties of feldspathic porcelain—Refer spotter questions

Table 1.13.1: Comparison of human, acrylic and porcelain teeth

Properties, units	Tooth enamel	Tooth dentin	Acrylic teeth	Feldspathic Porcelain
Density, gms/cc,	2.97	2.14	1.19	2.5
Proportional limit-PL, in MPa	224	148	27–45	
Compressive strength, CS in MPa	380	300	65–75	170
Tensile strength in MPa	10	51	55–65	25
Young's Modulus of elasticity $Y = Q = E = MPa$	80,000	18,000	2,500	70,000
Modulus of resilience $R = J/m^3$	0.55	0.94	0.32	
Surface hardness—KHN	340 or 300 VHN	68, or 62 VHN	16–20 Ht. cured	460, or 360 VHN
Thermal conductivity, $K = Cals/sec/cm^2/(°C/cm)$	0–0022	0.0016	0.006	0.0005
Coefficient of thermal expansion, COTE ppm/°C	11.4	8–6	80–120	9–12
Coefficient of diffusion $D = K/sp.$ heat × density, $mm^2/sec.$	0.469	0.183		

14. Dental Waxes (Auxiliary Materials)

Many verities of wax compositions are used as auxiliary materials in clinical and laboratory procedures for processing and preparing the pattern of moulds for fabrications of oral appliances. These are thermoplastic organic polymers, hydrocarbons of low molecular weights (400–4000), containing 15-55 carbon atoms, and their derivatives like esters, alcohols or free acids. Waxes of are classified according to their origins, (natural, plants, animal and synthetic), applications—(a) Pattern waxes (inlays, onlays, crowns, base plates), (b) Processing waxes (sticky, white, boxing, utility, blocking, beading, carving, etc.) (c) Impression waxes.

14-1. Dental waxes have temperature dependent COTE, in the ranges in ppm/°C:
 (a) 8.3–11.4   (b) 25–55
 (c) 81–120   (d) 250–400

14-2. Dental waxes have softening range of temperatures in °C:
 (a) 37–75   (b) 80–100
 (c) 110–120   (d) 135–150

14-3. When the temperature of dental waxes rises, following properties decrease:
 (a) Flow   (b) COTE.
 (c) Modulus of elasticity   (d) Flexibility

14-4. Distortion (wax memory) of dental waxes is due to:
 (a) Low thermal conductivity   (b) High COTE
 (c) None   (d) Both

14-5. Base plate dental wax is used for:
 (a) Pattern making   (b) Processing
 (c) Denture bases   (d) Denture repairing procedure

14-6. Dental sticky wax (model cement) is used for:
 (a) Pattern making   (b) Processing
 (c) Denture bases   (d) Denture repairing procedure

14-7. Inlay wax is used for:
 (a) Pattern making   (b) Cast-crowns
 (c) Denture bases   (d) Denture repairing procedure

14-8. Base plate dental wax mainly contains:
 (a) Bees' wax   (b) Paraffin wax
 (c) Ceresin wax   (d) Carnauba wax

14-9. Dental inlay pattern wax mainly contains:
 (a) Bees' wax   (b) Paraffin wax
 (c) Carnauba wax   (d) Ceresin wax

14-10. Dental inlay pattern waxes should have:
(a) No flaking or chipping while carving
(b) Flow >70% at 45°C.
(c) High thermal conductivity and low COTE
(d) All of the above

14-11. Distortion of wax patterns by relaxation of internal stresses is due to:
(a) Inhomogeneous softening and poor bonding of incremental layers
(b) Low thermal conduction
(c) High COTE
(d) All of the above

14-12. Disadvantage of direct pattern technique:
(a) Difficult to do carving
(b) Thermal shrinkage
(c) Distortion while dislodging
(d) All of the above

14-13. Disadvantage of indirect pattern technique is:
(a) Dimensional changes of dies
(b) Thermal shrinkage of impression
(b) Distortion while dislodging
(d) All of the above

14-14. Inlay wax pattern shrinkage in direct or indirect techniques is about:
(a) Negligible   (b) 0.3–0.4%
(c) 1.2–1.4%   (d) 2.3–2.5%

15. Casting Investments (Auxiliary Materials)

These are auxiliary refractory mould materials used for embedding the prepared wax patterns and thereby, obtaining the corresponding mould in the lost-wax casting technique, initiated by Taggart in 1907. This technique involves compensation of casting shrinkages by setting and thermal expansions of investments, etc.

15-1. Requirements of dental casting investment materials are large:
(a) Thermal expansion   (b) Setting expansion
(c) Porosity   (d) All of the above

15-2. Highest thermal expansion for refractory material is for:
(a) Cristobalite
(b) Amorphous quartz
(c) Crystalline quartz
(d) Tridymite

15-3. Type one investment material is used for:
(a) Brazing
(b) Large RPD casting
(c) Small castings with NSE
(d) Small castings with HSE

15-4. Common dental casting investment material now used is:
(a) Silica-bonded   (b) Gypsum-bonded
(c) Phosphate-bonded   (d) Resin-bonded

15-5. Thermal expansion of PBI investment materials is increased by:
(a) Increasing W/P
(b) Adding more colloidal silica
(c) Adding fluxes
(d) Lowering temperature

15-6. Phosphate bonded investment has inadequate:
(a) Thermal stability   (b) Strength
(c) Porosity   (d) All of the above

15-7. Refractory material of PBI for casting PBM alloys is:
(a) Amorphous quartz   (b) Crystalline quartz
(c) Cristobalite   (d) Alumina + zirconia

15-8. Alloy casting shrinkage is due to:
(a) Wax shrinkage   (b) Alloy shrinkages
(c) Both   (d) None

15-9. Wax pattern shrinkage in indirect technique is about:
(a) 0.4%   (b) 1.0%
(c) 1.8%   (d) 2.6%

15-10. **Alloy shrinkage for high fusing PBM alloys is about:**
(a) 1.4% (b) 2.3%
(c) 8.6% (d) 11.4%

15-11. **Alloy shrinkage for high fusing PBM alloys is more due to:**
(a) Higher fusion temperature (b) Lower density
(c) lower flexibility (d) Passivation

15-12. **Casting shrinkage is compensated by increasing:**
(a) Setting expansion of investment
(b) Thermal expansion of investment
(c) Colloidal silica liquid
(d) All of these

15-13. **Gypsum bonded investment has:**
(a) Adequate porosity
(b) Compressive strength >4.8 MPa in 2 hr
(c) Lack of porosity
(d) High thermal stability

15-14. **Phosphate bonded investment has:**
(a) Lack of porosity
(b) Compressive strength >4.8 MPa in 2 hrs
(c) High thermal stability
(d) All of the above

15-15. **Large expansion of PBI is obtained by using:**
(a) Setting expansions
(b) Thermal expansion
(c) More colloidal silica liquid
(d) All of the above

15-16. **Main disadvantages of phosphate bonded investments is:**
(a) Lack of porosity
(b) Compressive strength >4.8 MPa in 2 hrs
(c) Thermal stability
(d) All of the above

15-17. **Lack of porosity disadvantage of PBI is remedied by using:**
(a) Vent sprues (b) Thin long sprue
(c) Thick short sprues (d) Ring liners

15-18. Divestment technique is used to minimise:
(a) Casting shrinkages
(b) Distortion of large castings
(c) Incomplete castings
(d) Microporosities

15-19. PBM Alloy castings should be cooled slowly to:
(a) Increase corrosion resistance
(b) Control carbide precipitation, i.e. mechanical properties
(c) Homogenise
(d) Improve polishability

15-20. Silica-bonded investment is not popular due to:
(a) Complicated investing technique
(b) Lack of porosity
(c) Evolution of combustible alcohol vapour
(d) All of the above

15-21. Investment refractory material for titanium alloy castings, contain:
(a) Alumina + Zircona + MgO
(b) Amorphous quartz
(c) Cristobalite
(d) Tridymite

15-22. Investment materials for soldering should have:
(a) Large expansion
(b) High strength
(c) Least dimensional change
(d) Good abrasive resistance

16. Solidification of Metals and Alloys (Metallurgy)

Metallurgy refers to the study of a very important branch of science and technologies applied in the fabrications of many permanent oral appliances and instruments in dentistry, machines and machine parts used in all industries, domestic appliances, etc., in almost every fields.

Metals are defined as hard, opaque, lustrous chemical substances, having good thermal and electrical conductivities and reflecting light from polished surfaces, etc. More than 85 elements are metals!

16-1. The most important characteristics of metals is:
(a) Good thermal and electrical conductor
(b) Free electrons-metallic-bonding of atoms
(c) Form +ve ions in solution
(d) All of the above

16-2. The law of cooling, "rate of cooling is directly proportional to the temperature difference between the hot body and the surroundings" was stated by:
(a) Archimedes
(b) Newton
(c) Einstein
(d) Doppler

16-3. Metals solidify by:
(a) Super cooling
(b) Nucleation
(b) Dendrites and grain formation
(d) All of the above

16-4. Technique used to get finer grains is by:
(a) Heterogeneous nucleation
(b) Homogeneous nucleation
(c) Smaller super cooling
(d) Slow cooling

16-5. When large volume of liquid metal is solidified it forms crystals:
(a) Equi-axed (b) Fibrous
(c) Thin platelets (d) Irregular

16-6. The crystal-grains in small dental castings are:
(a) Radial (b) Columnar
(c) Irregular shape (d) Thin platelets

16-7. Purpose of alloying metals is to get desired properties:
(a) Biocompatibility, corrosion resistance
(b) Physical, mechanical
(c) Thermal
(d) All of these

16-8. Hume-Rothery conditions (criteria) for alloying, i.e. solid solubility:
(a) Atomic size difference should be <15%
(b) Valency must be same
(c) Should be similar lattice structures
(d) All of the above

16-9. Criteria to form solid solution is that they should have same or close:
(a) Atomic size
(b) Fusion temperatures
(c) Densities
(d) None of these

16-10. Which metal cannot dissolve in pure gold?
(a) Copper   (b) Zinc
(c) Platinum   (d) Silver

16-11. Solid solutions have:
(a) Higher ductility and malleability
(b) Higher fusion temperatures
(c) Range of fusion temperatures
(d) Lower slip-resistance-strength

16-12. Types of solid solutions:
(a) Substitutional   (b) Disordered, and ordered
(c) Interstitial   (d) All of the above

16-13. Terms related to alloys (or define each term):
(a) Equilibrium-phase   (b) Alloy-system
(c) Solvent, solute, solid solution   (d) All of these

16-14. Liquid and solid phases are present:
(a) Above liquidus
(b) Below solidus
(c) Between liquidus and solidus
(d) Below eutectic temperature

16-15. Cored (brittle inhomogeneous) cast structure is homogenised at:
(a) Half of its melting temperature in degree Kelvin
(b) Slightly below solidus for long time
(c) Between 375°C and 400°C
(d) At 779°C

16-16. As-cast alloys have:
    (a) Fibrous structure
    (b) Stress-free crystals with lattice defects
    (c) Strained grains
    (d) Ordered phases

16-17. Wrought alloys have:
    (a) Equi-axial crystal structure
    (b) Stress-free crystals with lattice
    (c) Strained distorted grains
    (d) Ordered phases

16-18. Solubility of copper in silver at eutectic temperature (779°C) is:
    (a) 5%   (b) 8.8%
    (c) 28%   (d) 92%

16-19. Solubility of silver in copper at eutectic temperature (779°C) is:
    (a) 5%   (b) 8.0%
    (c) 28%   (d) 92%

16-20. Silver-copper eutectic alloy has:
    (a) Alternate layers of alpha and beta solid solutions
    (b) Alpha solid solution
    (c) Beta solid solution
    (d) Disordered structure

16-21. Age hardening of alloys refers to:
    (a) Precipitation of super-saturated solute atoms
    (b) Precipitation of distorted phases
    (c) Martensitic structure
    (d) Eutectic alloys

16-22. Silver-copper eutectic atomised alloy is used:
    (a) For grain refinement
    (b) In admix silver amalgam alloy
    (b) In noble metal castings
    (d) None of these

16-23. Example for peritectic transformation, i.e. Liquid + disordered phase → ordered new phase refers to the alloy systems of:
    (a) Pd-Ag   (b) Ag-Sn
    (c) Au-Cu   (d) Ag-Cu

16-24. Gold-copper system phase-diagram is used to study:
(a) Solidification temperature ranges
(b) Disorder-order transformations
(c) Softening (solution), hardening heat-treatment techniques
(d) All of the above

16-25. Precipitation hardening of gold alloys takes place when copper present by weight % is:
(a) < 15% (b) 15–35%
(c) 40–70% (d) >85%

16-26. Precipitation hardening of cast gold alloys takes place when gold and copper alloy lattice is transformed into:
(a) Disordered fcc (b) Ordered fcc
(c) Ordered fct (d) Martensite

16-27. Softening or solution heat-treatments is done by heating the cast gold alloys to:
(a) Slightly below solidus for some time and quenching
(b) 375–400°C and slowly cooling
(c) 100°C for 24 hrs
(d) Half of its melting temperature in degree Kelvin for 8 min

16-28. Hardening heat-treatment is done by heating the gold alloy casts to:
(a) Slightly below solidus for some time and quenching
(b) 375–400°C for about 10 min and cool
(c) 100°C for 24 hrs
(d) Half of its melting temperature for 8 min

16-29. Binary alloys have:
(a) Simplest constitutional phase diagrams
(b) Two metals like Pd-Ag Au-Cu. Ag-Cu, etc.
(c) Disordered or ordered lattice structures
(d) All of the above

16-30. Intermetallic alloys:
(a) Are formed by chemical affinities in liquid states
(b) Have ordered lattices
(c) Have different properties
(d) All of the above

16-31. Equillibrium phase diagrams are used for controlling:
  (a) Melting temperature ranges
  (b) Micro-structure
  (c) Mechanical properties by heat treatments
  (d) All of the above

17. Dental Casting Alloys

Detailed knowledge of all the properties of various casting alloys and the alloying properties of their components is required for dentists to select the most suitable materials, and for technicians to adopt the appropriate fabrication techniques.

For approximate compositions, functions and properties of HN,N, and PBM alloys refer to Tables 1.17.1 to 1.17.5 given at the end.

17-1. Predominantly base metal (PBM) dental casting alloys are used for casting RPDs since the year:
  (a) 1907
  (b) 1933
  (c) 1984
  (d) 2002

17-2. Dental casting high noble metal alloys should have:
  (a) Noble metals >25%
  (b) Noble metals 0–25%
  (c) Gold >40% and noble metals >60%
  (d) Only gold and titanium

17-3. Dental casting noble metal alloys should have:
  (a) Noble metals >25%
  (b) Noble metals 0–25%
  (c) Gold >40% and noble metals >60%
  (d) Only gold and titanium

17-4. Dental casting predominantly base metal (PBM) alloys should have:
  (a) Noble metals >25%
  (b) Noble metals 0–25%
  (c) Gold >40% and noble metals >60%
  (d) Only gold and titanium

17-5. Dental casting alloys should be biocompatible, corrosion resistant and noncarcinogenic since they are required:
(a) In the mouth for long time
(b) To withstand large masticating forces
(c) Resist abrasion
(d) For aesthetics

17-6. Casting alloys should have high yield strength to resist:
(a) Permanent deformations (b) Elastic deformations
(c) Fractures   (d) Abrasions

17-7. Casting alloys should have high modulus of elasticity to resist:
(a) Any deformations   (b) Permanent deformations
(c) Fractures   (d) Abrasion

17-8. Casting alloys should have high modulus of resilience to:
(a) Resist permanent deformations
(b) Absorb deforming energies
(c) Have long life
(d) Resist fracture and abrasion

17-9. Casting alloys should have high fatigue strength or endurance limit to:
(a) Resist permanent deformations
(b) Absorb deforming energies
(c) Resist abrasions
(d) Have long life without fractures

17-10. Casting alloys should have high ultimate strengths to:
(a) Resist permanent deformation
(b) Absorb deforming energies
(c) Have long life
(d) Resist fractures

17-11. Casting alloys should have surface hardness:
(a) Low, for easy polishing
(b) Same as enamel
(c) High, for resisting abrasion
(d) All of the above

17-12. According to recent classifications, type 2, dental casting alloys should have minimum yield strength in MPa:
(a) 80　　　　　　　　　　(b) 180
(c) 270　　　　　　　　　(d) 360

17-13. According to recent classifications, type 3 dental casting alloys should have minimum percentage elongation:
(a) 18　　　　　　　　　　(b) 10
(c) 5　　　　　　　　　　　(d) 3

17-14. Type 3 hard-casting alloys are used for:
(a) Inlays at nonstress acting areas
(b) RPD frame works
(c) Thick crowns
(d) Crowns and bridges at high stress bearing areas

17-15. Predominantly base metal alloys contain major metal:
(a) Palladium or silver
(b) Chromium with cobalt or nickel, titanium
(c) Gold
(d) Copper

17-16. Gold alloy-916 fine refers to:
(a) 22 Karat gold alloy
(b) 91.6% gold
(c) 916 parts of gold in 1000 parts of alloy
(d) Any one

17-17. Addition of more copper in gold alloys increase:
(a) Corrosion resistance　　(b) Ductility
(c) Fusion temperature　　　(d) Strength, hardness

17-18. Addition of more silver in gold alloys increases:
(a) Corrosion resistance　(b) Ductility
(c) Fusion temperature　　(d) Strength and yellowness

17-19. Addition of more platinum or palladium to gold alloys:
(a) Increase fusion temperature and strength
(b) Decrease COTE
(c) Cause whitening
(d) All of the above

17-20. Zinc in gold alloys acts as:
(a) Surface hardener   (b) Scavenger
(c) Grain refiner   (d) Hardener

17-21. Copper in gold alloys causes hardness by:
(a) Solution hardening
(b) Precipitation of Au-Cu-phase
(c) Both
(d) None

17-22. Iridium has:
(a) High density = 22-5 gm/cc, and MP = 2454°C
(b) Low COTE = 6.8 ppm/°C
(c) Grain refining ability
(d) All of the above

17-23. Amount of gold in HN casting alloys is:
(a) 10–25%   (b) 40–80%
(c) 5–60%   (d) 1–4%

17-24. Amount of silver in HN alloys is:
(a) 10–25%   (b) 40–80%
(c) 5–60%   (d) 1–4%

17-25. Amount of palladium in noble alloys is:
(a) 10–25%   (b) 40–70%
(c) 5–60%   (d) 1–4%

17-26. Amount of silver in noble alloys is:
(a) 10–25%   (b) 40–70%
(c) 5–60%   (d) 1–4%

17-27. High noble and noble metal-ceramic alloys should have:
(a) Slightly miss-matched COTE
(b) Good bonding with ceramic
(c) Higher fusion temperature
(d) All of the above

17-28. Fusion temperatures of HN and N metal-ceramic alloys can be raised by adding more:
(a) Noble metals   (b) Pt or Pd
(c) Silver   (d) Chromium or copper

17-29. **COTE of HN and N metal-ceramic alloys can be lowered by adding more:**
(a) Noble metals
(b) Pt or Pd
(c) Silver
(d) Chromium

17-30. **PBM alloys are classified according to:**
(a) Applications
(b) Compositions
(c) Fusion temperatures
(d) All of the above

17-31. **Passivating metal in PBM alloys is:**
(a) Chromium
(b) Nickel
(c) Cobalt
(d) Beryllium

17-32. **Chromium is mainly used in PBM alloys to increase:**
(a) Strength
(b) Fusion temp
(c) Corrosion resistance
(d) Hardness

17-33. **Carbon 1–2% is used in PBM alloys to increase:**
(a) Strength
(b) Fusion temp
(c) Hardness
(d) Corrosion resistance

17-34. **Strength of cast PBM alloys is controlled by:**
(a) Carbide precipitation types—lamellar, island, etc.
(b) Rate of cooling
(a) Compositions
(d) All of the above

17-35. **Cobalt or nickel are mainly used in PBM alloys to increase:**
(a) Strength
(b) Hardness
(c) Fusion temperature
(d) All of the above

17-36. **Compared to Co alloys, Ni-alloys have higher:**
(a) Rigidity
(b) Fusion temperatures
(c) Hardness
(d) Percentage elongation

17-37. **Which of these has highest melting temperature?**
(a) Gold
(b) Platinum
(c) Silver
(d) Palladium

17-38. **Which of these has lowest melting temperature?**
(a) Gold
(b) Platinum
(c) Silver
(d) Palladium

17-39. Any Cr-Co-Ni, PBM casting alloy varieties should contain:
(a) Cr+ C   (b) Co+ Ni
(c) Cr+ Ni   (d) Cr+Be

17-40. PB investment is used in casting of PBM alloy as it has:
(a) High thermal stability   (b) High surface hardness
(c) Adhesion to castings   (d) Less porosity

17-41. Induction heating is used to melt, PBM alloys, as it has high:
(a) Fusion temperature
(b) Surface hardness
(c) Thermal stability
(d) Difficult to polish by abrasion

17-42. Electropolishing is used for PBM cast alloys as it has high:
(a) Thermal stability
(b) Strength
(c) Corrosion resistance
(d) Surface hardness

17-43. Technique (bronze) alloy-Japanese gold is not used for casting, since it has:
(a) Al-Cu-zinc   (b) Low strength
(c) Low corrosion resistance   (d) All of the above

Tables 1.17.1: Properties of alloying metals used in dentistry

Metal	Crystal structure	At. No.	Mass No.	Sp. gravity	COTE. ppm/°C	Melt. Temp. °C
Hg	rhombic	80	201	13.59	61.25	—38
Au	fcc	79	197	19.3	14.2	1063
Pt	fcc	78	195	21.5	8. 9	1769
Ir	fcc	77	192	22.5	6.8	2454
Os	hcp	76	190	22.48	7.0	3027
Sn	scc/bcc	50	119	7.3	40	232

(Contd.)

Tables 1.17.1: Properties of alloying metals used in dentistry *(Contd.)*

Metal	Crystal structure	At. No.	Mass No.	Sp. gravity	COTE. ppm/°C	Melt. Temp. °C
In	bcc/tetra	49	115	7.3	33	156
Cd	hcp	48	112	8.65	30	321
Ag	fcc	47	108	10.5	19.7	961
Pd	fcc	46	106	12	12.8	1552
Rh	fcc	45	103	12.44	11.2	1,927
Ru	hcp	44	101	12.4	13	2,247
Ge	scc/diamond	32	73	5.4	7.6	937
Ga	fcc/orthorho.	31	70	5.95	18	30
Zn	hcp	30	66	7.1	39.7	420 (BP,907)
Cu	fcc	29	64	8.93	16.5	1083
Ni	fcc	28	59	8.9	18.3	1453
Co	hcp/fcc/690°C	27	58	8.9	17.8	1492
Fe	bcc/-900°C-fcc/ 1390°C-bcc	26	56	7.87	13-15	1435
Mn	cubic	25	55	7.44	22	1244
Cr	bcc	24	52	7.2	8.4	1887
V	bcc	23	51	6.1	8	1887
Ti	hcp/885°C-bcc	22	48	4-54	8.6	1675
Si	cubic	14	28	2.3	7.1	14 = 7
Al	rhombic	13	27	2.7	7.6	660
C	cubic/graph/ diamond	6	12	2.3	1.6	>3500
O	rhombic	8	16	0.000133		−218.3
He	hcp/cubic	2	4	0.000166		−272
H	hcp/cubic	1	1	0.000089		−258.9

Noble metals (and their atomic numbers) used in dental casting alloys: Gold—79, platinum—78, iridium—77, osmium—76, *Silver—47(semi?),* palladium—46, rhodium—45, ruthenium—44

Table 1.17.2: Approximate compositions and alloying properties of high noble and noble casting alloys

Components	High noble-Au-alloys-yellow or white	Noble-Pd or Ag-alloys-white	Functions
Gold	40–80%	0–40%	Increases corrosion resist, and strength
Silver	10–25%	40–70%	Increases-strength, decreases-MP
Copper	6–15%	8–14%	Soln + Pptn. hardener, decreases MP, corrosion resist
Palladium or P	1–4%	5-60%	Increases strength, MP decreases COTE
Ga, Zn, In Ir	Trace	Trace	Scavengers, grain refiner

Table 1.17.3: Approximate properties of HN and N metal casting alloys (Types 1–4)

Properties	Softened by quenching or annealing	Heat hardened
Yield strength at 2% offset	100–430 (MPa)	270–580 (MPa)
Surface hardness	60–180 (VHN)	180–270 (VHN)
Elongation at fracture	35–39 %	6–20 %
Modulus of elasticity	90,000–110,000 (MPa)	Same
Biocompatibility	Excellent	Good

Table 1.17.4: Approximate properties of metal-ceramic alloys

Properties	High noble	Noble	PBM alloys
Corrosion. Resistance,	Excellent	Very good	Adequate
Density gm/cc,	14–18	10–12	8–9
Yield strength in MPa	450–680	460–500	500–700
Surface hardness-(softened) VHN	180–220	190–120	250–350
Elastic modulus-MPa	100,000	90,000	180,000–220,000
Elongation at fracture	5–20%	10–30%	2–8%
Fusion temp range °C	950–1050	1150–1300	1275–1350

Table 1.17.5: Approximate properties of predominantly base metal (PBM) dental casting alloys

Alloys	YS. in MPa	UTS, in MPa	Elongation min %	S,H. in VHN	Q,E- GPa	MP in °C middle of ranges
Cr-Co (Vitallium)	700	870	1.6	430	225	1410
Cr-Ni (Ticonium)	680	800	4.0	300	180	1275
Cr-Co- Ni (Jelenko)	500	700	8.0	260	200	1350
Hardened-type 4-gold alloys	490	775	7	265	90	960

18. Casting Procedure and Defects

Lost-wax casting procedure (Taggart, 1907) is quite complicated and time consuming. Unless all the precautions are meticulously taken care of, it is impossible to get precisely fitting defect less appliances. Main defects are, distortion, discoloration, surface irregularities-roughness, internal porosities, incomplete castings, fins, etc. Varieties of casting machines involve centrifugal force, compression, vacuum suction, etc., casting principles. Alloys are melted by different gas flames, electric arc or resistance, induction heating, etc., methods. Technician should have good theoretical knowledge and training.

18-1. Casting wax patterns are usually made from:
    (a) Inlay wax rods   (b) Modeling wax
    (c) Carving wax   (d) Sticky wax

18-2. Type 2 inlay wax is used for:
    (a) Indirect technique   (b) Direct technique
    (c) Vent sprue   (d) Preformed patterns

18-3. Sprue former is prepared from:
    (a) Inlay wax rods, sprue wax role
    (b) Steel-wire
    (c) Composite resins
    (d) Cross-linked PMMA

18-4. Diameter of sprues should be about:
    (a) Thinnest part of pattern
    (b) >thickest part of pattern
    (c) Exactly = 1.5 mm
    (d) 4.5 mm

18-5. Too long and very thin sprues result in:
    (a) Rough surface   (b) Incomplete castings
    (c) Pin-hole porosities   (d) Fins

18-6. Wax pattern is coated with a surfactant solution to:
    (a) Get wetted by investment mix
    (b) Increase its stiffness
    (c) Melt easily
    (d) Compensate casting shrinkages

18-7. **Too short or very thick sprues result in:**
(a) Rough surface
(b) Incomplete castings
(c) Pin-hole porosities
(d) Back pressure porosity

18-8. **The sprue is to be fixed to wax pattern inclined to occlusal surface at:**
(a) 0°   (b) 45°
(c) 37°C   (d) 90°

18-9. **Wetted ring liners are used to provide:**
(a) Adequate lateral expansion
(b) Extra water for HSE
(c) Easiness for devesting
(d) All of the above

18-10. **Method of mixing and investing is done by:**
(a) Hand   (b) Vacuum
(c) Mechanical   (d) Any

18-11. **Die-investing of large wax patterns is to reduce:**
(a) Internal porosities   (b) Incomplete castings
(c) Distortions   (d) Air inclusions

18-12. **Vent-sprue is required for PBI to reduce:**
(a) Internal porosities   (b) Back pressure porosity
(c) Air inclusions   (d) Distortions

18-13. **Wax burn-out after investing should be done:**
(a) Immediately   (b) After 30 min
(c) After 2 hrs   (d) On complete drying

18-14. **Rapid, prolonged and overheating of investment cause:**
(a) Fracture of investment   (b) Rough surface
(c) Fins   (d) All of the above

18-15. **Melting of high fusing alloys, nowadays, is done using:**
(a) Gas-torch-flame
(b) Oxy-acetylene flame
(c) Laser beam
(d) Induction heating technique

18-16. **Alloy liquid temperature while casting should be:**
  (a) Below liquidus
  (b) Just above solidus
  (c) 100°C above liquidus
  (d) Between solidus and liquidus

18-17. **If the temperature of alloy liquid is very high, while casting, it causes:**
  (a) Rough surface, hot spot porosity
  (b) Incomplete casting
  (c) Fins
  (d) Air inclusions

18-18. **If the temperature of alloy liquid, while casting, is too low, it causes:**
  (a) Rough surface
  (b) Incomplete casting
  (c) Fins
  (d) Air inclusions

18-19. **Quenching of HN and N cast immediately, causes:**
  (a) Precipitation of super-lattice
  (b) Increases surface hardness
  (c) Solution hardening or Soft condition
  (d) Brittleness

18-20. **The finished gold alloy casting is subjected to heat treatments for:**
  (a) Annealing, homogenizing
  (b) Solution hardening
  (c) Super-lattice precipitation
  (d) All of the above

CASTING DEFECTS

18-21. **Distortion of shape of cast is due to:**
  (a) Mishandling of wax pattern
  (b) Incomplete wax burn-out
  (c) Thin sprue
  (d) Inadequate casting shrinkage compensation

18-22. **Distortion of shape and size cause:**
  (a) Discoloration
  (b) Misfit
  (c) Nodules
  (d) Decrease of strength

18-23. **Discolorations of HN alloy castings is due to:**
(a) SO_2 gas of overheated GBI
(b) NH_3 gas of PBI
(c) Ethyl alcohol vapours
(d) Overheated alloy liquid

18-24. **Nodules on the cast surface are caused by:**
(a) Coarse investment particles
(b) Improper wetting of wax pattern
(c) Rapid wax burnout
(d) Vacuum-investing

18-25. **Rough cast surfaces are due to:**
(a) Coarse investment particles
(b) Inadequate mixing of investment
(c) Rapid wax burn-out
(d) All of the above

18-26. **Sudden solidification of casting alloy liquid causes shrinkage porosities as:**
(a) Irregular micro-voids
(b) Regular pin-holes
(c) Hot-spot voids
(d) Large spherical voids

18-27. **Localized shrinkage porosity can be avoided by using:**
(a) Higher casting force
(b) Lowering investment temperature
(c) Higher temperature of casting liquid
(d) A reservoir near the pattern

18-28. **Pin-hole porosity is due to:**
(a) Solidification shrinkage
(b) Release of gases absorbed in alloy liquid
(c) Mixing of air in liquid while casting
(d) Hot-spot of investment

18-29. **Back-pressure porosity is caused by:**
(a) High casting force
(b) Air trapped in the mould
(c) Air inclusions in alloy liquid
(d) Porous investment

18-30. Back-pressure porosity can be avoided by:
(a) Higher casting force
(b) Fixing a vent sprue
(c) Using a larger reservoir
(d) Using more ring-liners

18-31. Incomplete casting is due to:
(a) Insufficient alloy liquid filling the mould
(b) Larger reservoir
(c) Solidification shrinkage
(d) Short-thick sprue

18-32. Fins on the cast-surfaces are caused due to:
(a) Porous investment
(b) Silica-bonded investment
(c) Fracture of investment
(d) Low casting temperature

18-33. To avoid all the casting fabrication defects, use:
(a) Induction melting   (b) Vacuum casting
(c) Centrifugal casting   (d) CAD-CAM technique

18-34. Dental casting titanium is:
(a) α-Ti   (b) β-Ti
(c) TMA (Ti-Mo-Zr)   (d) Ni-Ti

19-35. Refractory material for casting of titanium and its alloys is:
(a) Amorphous quartz   (b) $Al_2O_3 + ZrO_2$
(c) Cristobalite   (d) Tridymite

18-36. Centrifugal force alone is not adequate for casting titanium since it has:
(a) Low density = 4.51 gm/cc
(b) Allotropic forms
(c) Oxide surface layer
(d) High fusion temperature

18-37. Casting technique for titanium involves:
(a) Induction-melting
(b) Centrifugal machine and vacuum casting
(d) Pressure cum suction-device
(d) All of the above

18-38. Advantages of CAD-CAM technique:
    (a) Non-porous best ceramics or castings can be selected
    (b) Less time consuming and less dentist's fatigue
    (c) Chair-side procedure
    (d) All of the above

18-39. Alternatives to the complicated casting techniques:
    (a) Chair-side, CAD-CAM technique and copy-milling
    (b) Electroforming
    (c) Sintering of burnished foil
    (d) Any of these

19. Wrought Alloys

As-cast alloys are very rarely used directly. They contain stress-free equi-axial crystals and many lattice defects, which make them soft, ductile and malleable. These are subjected to many repeated deformations (by drawing, hammering, forging, etc.). The lattice defects move to the grain boundaries or inter dendritic spaces, causing work or strain hardening which increases strength, decreases ductility, malleability, and corrosion resistances. Annealing heat treatment is given to avoid distortion, and retain the desired shapes and properties.

19-1. As-cast alloys have:
    (a) Stress-free crystals, ductility and malleability
    (b) Dendrites with lattice defects
    (c) Equi-axial grains with grain boundaries
    (d) All of the above

19-2. Metal alloys have high strengths if:
    (a) Many lattice defects and voids are present
    (b) Lattices structures are perfect
    (c) Density is high
    (d) Atomic number is high

19-3. Strength of as-cast alloy can be increased by:
    (a) Reducing lattices imperfections
    (b) Increasing slip resistance by solid solutions
    (c) Precipitations of solutes and new phases
    (d) All of the above

19-4. Mechanisms of increasing strength by raising slip resistance is by:
(a) Solution hardening
(b) Precipitations of solutes and super lattices
(c) Grain refinement
(d) Any one or all

19-5. Work-hardening refers to:
(a) Increase of slip resistance or hardness by repeated deformations
(b) Decrease of slip-resistance
(c) Precipitation hardening
(d) Solid solution formation

19-6. Shiffting the lattice defects to grain boundaries by deformation refers to:
(a) Tempering
(b) Annealing
(c) Work hardening
(d) Heat hardening

19-7. Cold-work increases:
(a) Strength and brittleness
(b) Ductility and malleability
(c) Corrosion resistance
(d) Fusion temperatures

19-8. Annealing of cold worked material is done at:
(a) Slightly below solidus
(b) 375°C for few min
(c) 779°C
(d) Half of its MP in degree Kelvin

19-9. Recovery-annealing heat treatment of wrought materials is required for:
(a) Increasing rigidity
(b) Raise abrasive resistance
(c) Relaxation of internal stresses
(d) Recrystallisation

19-10. Recrystallisation by annealing of ortho-wire appliances should not be done, since it:
(a) Gains corrosion resistance
(b) Becomes ductile

(c) Decreases mechanical properties by change in its fibrous to spherical grain structure

(d) None of these

19-11. Prolonged annealing causes grain growth which decreases:
(a) Strength   (b) Fusion temperature
(c) Ductility   (d) Malleability

20. Carbon-steels and Stainless Steels

Pure soft iron is a ductile, malleable metal, having high fusion temperature, 1527°C, density = 7.878 gm/cc. Its main allotropic forms are:

(a) Ferrite—α-iron-BCC, up to 768°C and is magnetic
(b) Ferrite—β-iron-BCC, up to 910°C.and is para-magnetic
(c) Austenite—γ-iron-FCC, up to 1400°C—nonmagnetic
(d) Austenite—δ-iron-above this, BCC—nonmagnetic

Very small amounts of carbon (sometimes as impurities) form very hard interstitial carbon-steel alloys of above verities. Susceptibility to high corrosion in moist atmosphere, etc., is remedied by addition of chromium, which is called stainless steels.

20-1. Cementite the hardest verity is:
(a) Iron carbide   (b) Pearlite steal
(c) Austenitic steel   (d) Martensite

20-2. Ferritic steel verity is:
(a) Alpha iron carbide   (b) Interstitial alloy
(c) Carbon <0.02%   (d) All of the above

20-3. Austenitic steel has:
(a) Carbon<2.03%   (b) Carbon >2.03%
(c) Least ductility   (d) Magnetic properties

20-4. Eutectoid-Pearlite steel has:
(a) Carbon = 0.8%
(b) Alternate layers of ferrite and cementite
(c) Transformed by slow cooling from austenite below 723°C
(d) All of the above

20-5. Martensitic steel is formed by:
(a) Eutectoid transformation
(b) Peritectic change
(c) Diffusion-less transformation of austenite
(d) All of the above

20-6. Chromium (11.5–27%) by stainless steel:
(a) Cause passivation
(b) Increase of melting temperature
(c) Depresses martensite formation temperature
(d) Lowers corrosion resistance

20-7. Nickel in austenitic or 18–8 stainless steel:
(a) Cause passivation
(b) Increase of melting temperature
(c) Lowers martensite formation temperature
(d) Lowers corrosion resistance

20-8. Ferritic stainless steel is mainly used for:
(a) Large sized parts in industries
(b) House-hold and dental instruments
(c) Hardened blades or teeth of cutting instruments
(d) Casting onlays

20-9. Austenitic 18–8 stainless steel is mainly used for:
(a) Large sized parts in industries
(b) House-hold and dental applications
(c) Hardened blades or teeth of cutting instruments
(d) Casting onlays

20-10. Martensitic stainless steel is mainly used for:
(a) For large sized parts in industries
(b) House-hold and dental applications
(c) Hardened blades or teeth of burs and cutting instruments
(d) Casting onlays

20-11. Hardness of steels is higher when:
(a) Carbon content is less
(b) More carbon, and martensite is formed
(c) Nickel content is lower
(d) Chromium is not added

20-12. Passivation of stainless steel refers to:
    (a) Increase of corrosion resistance by adding Cr
    (b) Decrease of melting temperature –ranges
    (c) Increase of COTE
    (d) Loss of corrosion resistance when heated

20-13. Sensitization of stainless steel refers to:
    (a) Increase of corrosion resistance
    (b) Arresting of diffusion of carbon by Niobium or Ti, Tn
    (c) Increase of COTE
    (d) Loss of corrosion resistance when heated

20-14. Corrosion resistance of austenitic stainless steel is retained temporarily at high temperatures by adding:
    (a) Niobium or Ti with tantalum
    (b) Nickel six times carbon
    (c) More carbon
    (d) None of these

20-15. Disadvantage of 18–8 stainless steel for denture base:
    (a) Lighter, due to thinness
    (b) Higher impact strength
    (c) Adaptation-fitting
    (d) High thermal conductivity

Table 1.20.1: Compositions of stainless steels in wt % (AISI series)

Varieties/AISI-Series		Chromium	Nickel	Carbon	Others + Fe
Ferritic,	400 BCC	11.5–27	0	0–0.2	Mn = 2 + Fe
Martensitic,	400 BCT	11.5–17	0–2.5	0.15–1.2	Mn = 2
Austenitic,	300 FCC	16–26	7–22	0–0.25	Mn = 2
18-8 stainless steel	302 FCC	18 (17–19)	8–10 (8)	0.15 (<0.17)	Mn = 2
Surgical	304 FCC	18–20	8-12	< 0.08	Mn = 2
Low carbon implants	316—L	16–18	10–14	<0.03	Mn = 2 Mo = 2–3

21. Materials used in Orthodontia

Orthodontia, dental speciality, refers to:

"The study of the growth of cranio-facial complex, i.e. the development of occlusion and masticatory apparatus," or to "the treatments like preventions, interceptions, corrections of malocclusions and other abnormalities, sometimes with surgeries for achieving maximum aesthetics and functional harmonies".

These are achieved by fabricating and using different types of force delivery mechanisms such as-active (removable, fixed, semi-fixed) and passive or reactive (functional, retention, habit-breaking) appliances.

21-1. Requirements of wire-materials for active appliances:
    (a) Biocompatibility, corrosion resistance
    (b) Low modulus of elasticity, high flexibility and resilience
    (c) Ability to solder and weld without recrystallisation
    (d) All of the above

21-2. Requirements of wire-materials for reactive appliances:
    (a) Biocompatibility and corrosion resistance
    (b) High modulus of elasticity, resilience and rigidity
    (c) Ability to solder and weld without recrystallization
    (d) All of the above

21-3. Most suitable wire materials (lowest modulus of elasticity) for active appliances is:
    (a) Elgilloy
    (b) 18–8 stainless steel
    (c) Nickel titanium
    (d) Pt-Au-P

21-4. Wire materials most suitable (highest modulus of elasticity) for reactive appliances is:
    (a) 18-8 stainless steel   (b) Beta titanium
    (c) Nickel titanium   (d) Alpha titanium

21-5. Micro-structure of grains of wrought orthodontic wires:
    (a) Platelet   (b) Equi-axial
    (c) Fibrous   (d) None of these

21-6. Thinner wires have higher strengths due to:
  (a) Greater work hardening
  (b) Finer fibrils microstructure
  (c) Both
  (d) None

21-7. Orthodontic-wires can be classified according to:
  (a) Nature of appliance—active/passive
  (b) Materials
  (c) Dispensing—shape, cross-section, tempering-soft ductile, high-tempered, etc.
  (d) Any

21-8. Orthodontic-wires are annealed to:
  (a) Avoid later distortions
  (b) Recover from internal stresses
  (c) Improve corrosion resistance
  (d) All of the above

21-9. Orthodontic-wires are tempered to:
  (a) Get suitable flexibility
  (b) Recover from internal stresses
  (c) Improve corrosion resistance
  (d) All of the above

21-10. 18–8 stainless steel orthodontic wires has advantage for reactive appliances due to its:
  (a) Rigidity
  (b) Low COTE
  (c) Good thermal conductivity
  (d) High fusion temperature

21-11. Passivation of stainless steel refers to:
  (a) Increasing of corrosion resistance
  (b) Decreasing melting temperature–range
  (c) Increase of COTE
  (d) Loss of corrosion resistance when heated

21-12. Sensitization of stainless steel refers to:
  (a) Loss of corrosion resistance during heating
  (b) Decreasing melting temperature–ranges
  (c) Increase of COTE
  (d) Retention of corrosion resistance when heated

21-13. **Corrosion resistance of 18-8 stainless steel at high temperatures is retained, i.e. temporarily stabilized by:**
   (a) Addition of niobium or Ti with tantalum six times carbon
   (b) Decreasing melting temperature
   (c) Decreasing COTE
   (d) Addition of cadmium

21-14. **Elgiloy (watch-spring) wire contains:**
   (a) Cr-Co-Be
   (b) Cr-Co-Ni-Fe
   (c) Pd-Gold-Pt
   (d) Ni-Ti

21-15. **Elgiloy (watch-spring) wire has properties similar to:**
   (a) Ni-Ti
   (b) CpTi
   (c) PGP
   (d) 18-8 stainless steel

21-16. **High noble-PGP (Pd + Au + Pt) wires have:**
   (a) Superelasticity
   (b) Elastic memory
   (c) Very low modulus of elasticity
   (d) High recrystallization temperatures

21-17. **When commercially pure α Ti is heated above 885°C, it:**
   (a) Changes from HCP martensite to β-Ti, bcc austenite
   (b) Loses corrosion resistance
   (c) Melts
   (d) Becomes more rigid

21-18. **Characteristic property of β-Ti, bcc austenite is:**
   (a) High UTS. and lower elastic modulus
   (b) Perfect weld ability
   (c) Large elastic-range
   (d) All of the above

21-19. TM alloy wire, (Ti = 79%, Mo = 11%, Zr = 6%, Sn = 4%) has properties similar to:

    (a) Cp-Ti, or β-Ti

    (b) 18-8 stainless steel

    (c) Ni-Ti

    (d) PGP(Pd-Au-Pt)

21-20. Elastic modulus of Ni-Ti wire in GPa is:

    (a) 41.4   (b) 71.7

    (c) 110   (d) 180

21-21. Characteristic property of Ni-Ti ortho-wire is:

    (a) High UTS and low elastic modulus

    (b) Thermal-shape memory due to twinning

    (c) Superelasticity

    (d) All of the above

21-22. Austenitic nickel-titanium becomes martensitic when:

    (a) Stressed or cooled below TTR

    (b) Heated above TTR

    (c) 42%-cobalt is added

    (d) It contains chromium

21-23. Disadvantage of nittinol arch wires is:

    (a) Lowest elastic modulus

    (b) Quick elastic recovery

    (c) Low density

    (d) Superelasticity

21-24. Recent experimental orthodontic wire is:

    (a) Teflon resin-coated Ni-Ti or β-Ti

    (b) Optiflex glass-fibre reinforced thermoplastic

    (c) Ti + V + Cr + Al + Sn alloy

    (d) All of the above

21-25. Mechanical properties of orthodontic wires depend on:

    (a) Thinness—greater work hardening

    (b) Tempering heat treatments

    (c) Compositions

    (d) All of the above

Table 1.21.1: Approximate comparative properties of orthodontic wires

Materials,	YS in MPa	UTS in MPa	Modulus of elasticity E in MPa	Mod of resilience $(YS)^2/2E$ J/m^3	Elastic-range YS/E Springback	Springi-ness = $10^{-6}/E$
18-8 stainless steel	1600	2100	180,000	6.94	0.00877	O.55
Elgilloy Cr + Co + Ni + Fe	1410	1700	184,000	5.402	0.00766	0.54
Ni-Ti (54% + 44%) + Cu or Co = 2%	430	1400	41,400	2.233	0.104	2.4
cpTi—β Ti, and TMA	930	1275	71,700	6,074	0.013	1.4
Pt-Au-Pd	1000	1200	110,000	4.54	0.009	0.91

22. Brazing—Soldering and Welding

Many metal-joining techniques are used in dentistry and industries to get larger devices from smaller components. These are soldering, brazing, welding, cast joining, etc. High technical skill is required to retain the best properties, while handling the heating devices, applications of fluxes and antifluxes, adjustments of gap distances, controlling microstructures of joints by time and temperatures, etc.

22-1. **The term, brazing is used when the liquidus temperature of solder is:**
   (a) Above 450°C
   (b) Below 450°C
   (c) Just above the solidus of components
   (d) Just below solidus of components

22-2. Ideally, brazers (hard solders) should have:
 (a) Lower melting temp, < 100°C from basis metals
 (b) High tensile strength > the components
 (c) High corrosion resistance and biocompatibility
 (d) All of the above

22-3. Soft solders (MP < 450°C) are not used in dentistry due to low:
 (a) Corrosion resistance (b) Strength
 (c) Surface hardness (d) All of the above

22-4. Gold solders have:
 (a) Liquidus temperature > 700°C
 (b) Fineness >650
 (c) Tensile strength > 430 MPa
 (d) All of the above

22-5. Silver solders contain:
 (a) Gold >40% (b) Silver 10–80%
 (c) Chromium 12% (d) Cadmium-43%

22-6. Free-flow solder refers to:
 (a) Low-viscosity and surface tension, molten solder, which wets and flows
 (b) High fusing solder
 (c) Low fusing solder, temperature 55°C, below solidus of basis metals
 (d) None

22-7. Easy-flow solder refers to:
 (a) Soft solder
 (b) Low-viscosity and surface tension, molten solder, which wets and flows
 (c) High fusing solder
 (d) Low fusing solder, temperature 55°C below solidus of basis metals

22-8. Microstructure of good soldered joints show:
 (a) Sharp boundary without diffusion of solder into the grains
 (b) Grain growth
 (c) Re-crystallization
 (d) Diffusion of molten solder into basis metals

22-9. **For adequate corrosion resistance, gold solders should have minimum gold content:**
   (a) 25%   (b) 40%
   (c) 650 fineness   (d) 22 Carats

22-10. **Soldering fluxes are used for:**
   (a) Wetting the basis metal surface
   (b) Increasing the melting temperature of solders
   (c) Preventing flow of molten solder
   (d) Enhancing oxide layer

22-11. **Type 2-fluoride containing soldering flux is used for soldering:**
   (a) Gold alloys
   (b) Silver alloys
   (c) Base metals
   (d) Ni-titanium

22-12. **Anti-fluxes (rouge or lead pencil markings) are used in soldering to:**
   (a) Limit flow of molten solder
   (b) Enhance flow
   (b) Reduce oxide-layer
   (d) Improve bond strength

22-13. **Propane and butane gas flames have temperatures:**
   (a) Inadequate to melt gold alloys
   (b) Inadequate for base metal alloys
   (c) Adequate for any-metal soldering
   (d) > 6,800°C

22-14. **Which gas-flame zone is suitable for soldering?**
   (a) Outer oxidising
   (b) Combustion
   (c) Inner gas + air mixing
   (d) Inner pale blue-reducing

22-15. **Disadvantage of free-hand soldering of large casts is:**
   (a) Distortions of appliances
   (b) Difficult to apply fluxes
   (c) Complicated technique
   (d) Time consuming

22-16. Soldering investment material should have:
(a) Strength > 4.8 MPa
(b) Adequate porosity
(c) Dimensional stability
(d) High corrosion resistance

22-17. Pitted solder joints occur due to:
(a) Gases absorbed by molten solder
(b) Gases released by basis metals
(c) Fluxes not applied
(d) Trapping of antifluxes

22-18. Electric-spot welding is done by localised quick melting of joining parts of components by:
(a) Electric current = 15–25 mA for 8–10 hrs
(b) AC or DC > 750 amps for 1/50 sec
(c) AC or DC of 50 amps for 18 min
(d) Induction heating

22-19. Weld-decay refers to failure of 18-8 stainless steel welding, due to:
(a) Inadequate melting   (b) Air-inclusion
(c) Passivation   (d) Sensitisation

22-20. Pre-brazing refers to:
(a) Cast-joining technique
(b) Casting to embedded alloys
(c) Brazing before ceramic veneering
(d) Brazing before finishing

22-21. Titanium-cast parts are best welded by:
(a) Electric-spot welding
(b) Oxy-acetylene gas
(c) Laser or plasma in an argon gas
(d) Infrared heat rays

22-22. Laser applications indicated in dentistry for:
Gingivectomy, gingivoplasty, gingival depigmentation, frenectomy and frenotomy, gingival troughing for crown-impressions, removal of gingival hypertrophy, leukoplakia, oral pepillectomies, pulpotomy, etc.

Advantages of laser applications:
(a) Dry bloodless, painless surgery
(b) Low mechanical trauma

(c) Minimum postoperative pain and swelling
(d) No pain or sedative injections
(e) Instant sterilization of surgical sites
(f) Minimum discomfort to the patiens

23. Tarnish and Corrosion

Verities of metallic fabrications are used in the patients' oral cavities, many times to serve for a long period. These should not undergo tarnish (discoloration-affecting aesthetics) and corrosion (degradations of surfaces). Knowledge of causes and remedies is required for selection of materials.

Tarnish is the discoloration of the surfaces of metallic appliances due to chemical action forming a thin surface film. Corrosion is the loss of materials from the surface, by chemical attacks on the surface particles. Tarnish is the fore-runner of corrosion. Dry and wet (electrolytic) corrosions cause degradation of the surfaces of appliances which are to be prevented.

23-1. Tarnishing of surfaces of restorations is due to:
(a) Galvanism   (b) Electrolytic dissolution
(c) Chromium   (d) Deposits and stains

23-2. Tarnishing of metallic appliances is due to:
(a) Internal stress relaxations
(b) Sensitization
(c) Rough surfaces
(d) Staining by foods and beverages

23-3. Dry corrosion takes place without contact to liquids due to:
(a) Stress relaxations
(b) Dissimilar metals coming into contact
(c) Electrolytes
(d) Formation of oxide films on metal surfaces

23-4. Example for electrochemical or wet corrosion is:
(a) Galvanic corrosion
(b) Heterogeneous compositions
(c) Concentration cell-crevice corrosion
(d) All of the above

23-5. Galvanic corrosion can be prevented by:
(a) Cavity varnishes
(b) Avoiding dissimilar alloys coming into contact
(c) Polishing the surface
(d) None of these

23-6. Galvanic shock can be prevented by:
(a) Applying insulating cement base
(d) Avoiding dissimilar alloys coming into contact
(c) Using same alloy to opposing teeth
(d) Any of these

23-7. Severely deformed areas of metallic appliances under go:
(a) Cell-corrosion
(b) Galvanic corrosion
(c) Stress or strain corrosion
(d) Inhomogeneous—alloy-corrosion

23-8. Cell corrosion is minimised by:
(a) Annealing   (b) Pickling
(c) Polishing   (d) Precipitation hardening

23-9. Stress corrosion can be remedied by:
(a) Passivation   (b) Annealing heat treatment
(c) Stabilisation   (d) Sensitisation

23-10. Corrosion can be measured by:
(a) Change in electrical resistance
(b) Corrosion-loss measurements
(c) Electro-chemical linear polarisation
(d) Any of the above

23-11. Methods of minimising tarnish and corrosion by:
(a) Maintaining oral hygiene
(b) Annealing of appliances
(c) Well-polishing
(d) Passivation of base metal-alloy
(e) Avoid prolonged and over-heating
(f) Quick soldering, welding and reduce their numbers
(g) Avoid base metals contacting hypochlorites
(h) Avoid contacts of dissimilar metals

24. Dental Implants

Dental implants can be defined as foreign biomaterials anchored to the jaw in order to reproduce an entire tooth, either as a single restoration, or as a support for removable or fixed partial dentures [or as a medical device], prepared from one or more biomaterials, intentionally placed within the body, totally or partially inserted in epithelial surface to assist normal functioning of the body. These should interact (bioactive) with the body tissues without producing harmful bio-hazardous effects.

Indications to dental implantations are: Motivation, good oral hygiene, and adequate bone structures, lengths, heights and contour for supporting desired sub-periosteal, transosteal or endosseous varieties.

Contraindications to dental implantations are: debility, uncontrollable diseases, diseases which are affected by implants, poor hygiene, sensitivity to implant materials, impossibility of prosthetic constructions.

24-1. Dental implant is a foreign bio-material device:
    (a) Anchored in the jaws
    (b) Fitted to the root canal
    (c) Cemented to the tooth crown
    (d) Seated on the edentulous region

24-2. Bio-activity refers to:
    (a) Bio-degradation
    (b) Undesired responses of materials in oral cavity
    (c) Osseointegrating property
    (d) Resisting corrosion

24-3. Requirements of implant materials:
    (a) Bio-activity   (b) High flexibility
    (c) Large elastic property   (d) Springiness

24-4. Requirements of implant materials:
    (a) Formation of strong osseointegrating interface
    (b) High flexibility
    (c) Large elastic deformations
    (d) Springiness

24-5. Requirements of implant materials:
(a) High flexibility
(b) Good surface texture
(c) Thermal and mechanical properties similar to bone
(d) Springiness

24-6. The most suitable bioactive material used for dental implants is:
(a) Noble metal alloys
(b) Pure gold
(c) 18-8 stainless steel
(d) Titanium or Ti-6Al-4V alloys

24-7. The material most suitable for dental implants is:
(a) Titanium or Ti-6Al-4V alloys
(b) Poly silicones
(c) Bio-glasses
(d) Inert ceramics like alumina or zirconia

24-8. The implants placed under periosteum over bony cortex is called:
(a) Transosteal
(b) Endosseous—endosteal
(c) Subperiosteal
(d) Epithelial

24-9. The implant partially submerged in alveolar of mandible is:
(a) Transosteal
(b) Endosseous—endosteal
(c) Subperiosteal
(d) Epithelial

24-10. The implant passing through alveolar bones is:
(a) Transosteal
(b) Endosseous—endosteal
(c) Subperiosteal
(d) Epithelial

24-11. The implant inserted into oral mucosa is called:
(a) Transosteal
(b) Endosseous—endosteal
(c) Subperiosteal
(d) Epithelial

24-12. For stronger implants, metal-bone bonding method used is, by:
(a) Forming thicker harder oxide layer
(b) Surface texturing
(c) Surface coating
(d) Any method

24-13. Metallic implants are surface coated with:
(a) Hydroxyapetite or tri-calcium phosphate
(b) Vinyl silanes
(c) Electrodeposition of gold
(d) Resin paints

24-14. Common intramobile element—IME, used for stress relief or shock absorption is:
(a) Graphite
(b) Bioglasses
(c) Poly oxy-methelene
(d) Titanium or Ti-6Al-4V alloys

25 Cutting, Abrasion and Finishing Mechanisms and Tools

Finishing of oral appliances involving, cutting, abrasion and polishing is to be done carefully to minimise, tarnishing, corrosion, irritation to soft tissues, and to maintain oral hygiene and best aesthetics. These procedures are performed with various instruments and technique.

Cutting of large unwanted portions of teeth, castings, oral appliances, etc. (for which compressive strengths are greater than the shearing strength), are done with hard regular shaped, sharp edged bladed instruments (knives, burs, etc.), first by applying large compressive force (greater than the proportional limits) on the work and then shearing to fracture and remove the shaving-pieces.

Abrasion is the removal of unwanted material from the surface by friction, grinding, or wearing, using large number of hard powdered particles, with irregularly shaped sharp-edges, directly or embedded to plane surfaces and rotating instruments, which are moved unidirectionally.

Final finishing to get smooth, glossy, reflecting micro-crystalline surface(Beilby layer) is achieved by polishing (with very fine hard particles in dry or slurry form, pressing and moving on the surface in multidirections), glazing or electro-polishing methods.

25-1. Purpose of finishing of oral appliances is to avail:
(a) Good aesthetics
(b) Resistance to tarnish and corrosion
(c) Better hygiene and less irritation to opposing tissues
(d) All of the above

25-2. Bulk reduction of appliances is done by:
(a) Regular bladed hand cutting or rotary instruments.
(b) Abrasions
(c) Glazing
(d) Polishing

25-3. The dental bur-head material is of:
(a) Alpha Titanium
(b) Hardened carbon steel
(c) Nickel titanium
(d) Elgilloy

25-4. The hardest cutting tool is of:
(a) Martensified carbon steel
(b) Tungsten carbide
(c) Silicon carbide
(d) Diamond points and discs

25-5. Dental cutting rotary burs can be classified according to:
(a) Bur materials and designs
(b) Rotating systems and speeds
(c) Clinical uses
(d) All these methods

25-6. Straight fissure steel bur is used to get tooth cavity's:
(a) Floor levelling and undercuts of cavity
(b) Width or size increasing
(c) Depth increasing
(d) Cavo-surface adjustment

25-7. **Round steel bur is used to get tooth cavity's:**
   (a) Floor levelling and undercuts of cavity
   (b) Width or size increasing
   (c) Depth increasing
   (d) Cavo-surface adjustment

25-8. **Inverted-cone steel bur is used to get tooth cavity's:**
   (a) Floor levelling and undercuts of cavity
   (b) Width or size increasing
   (c) Depth increasing
   (d) Cavo-surface adjustment

25-9. **Efficiency of cutting is higher, when:**
   (a) Rake angle is positive
   (b) Rake angle is negative
   (c) Tooth angle is larger
   (d) Number of teeth is less

25-10. **Efficiency of cutting of dental burs is LESS if:**
   (a) Speed or load are more
   (b) Rake angle is negative
   (b) Number of teeth is more
   (d) Tooth angle is smaller

25-11. **Rake-angle of steel bur is the angle between:**
   (a) Front and back of next tooth
   (b) Back of tooth and work surface
   (c) Front and back of same tooth
   (d) Front and radial line of tooth

25-12. **Tooth angle of steel bur is the angle between:**
   (a) Front and back of next tooth
   (b) Back of tooth and work surface
   (c) Front and back of same tooth
   (d) Front and radial line of tooth

25-13. **Clearance angle of steel bur is the angle between:**
   (a) Front and back of next tooth
   (b) Back of tooth and work surface
   (c) Front and back of same tooth
   (d) Front and radial line of tooth

25-14. Negative rake angled burs are used in dentistry due to:
(a) Lower heat generated and longer life
(b) Lower cutting efficiency
(c) More heat of cutting
(d) Easy to prepare

25-15. Chattering of burs during cavity preparation occurs due to:
(a) Eccentric mounting
(b) Run-out of teeth
(c) Inadequate lubrication
(d) All of these

25-16. Loss of material from surfaces or wearing can be due to:
(a) Chemical-erosion by acid-etching or corrosion
(b) Hard particles erosions by sand blasting, air abrasions
(c) Mechanical abrasion by hard particles
(d) All of these

25-17. Hardness of synthetic diamond abrasives in KHN is about:
(a) 800–820　　　　　　(b) 1,200–2,000
(c) 2,400–2,600　　　　(d) >5,000

25-18. Hardness of sand, silica, quartz abrasives in KHN is about:
(a) 800–820　　　　　　(b) 1,200–2,000
(c) 2,400–2,600　　　　(d) >5,000

25-19. Hardness of Si, B, W. Carbide abrasives in KHN are about:
(a) 800–820　　　　　　(b) 1,200–2,000
(c) 2,400–2,600　　　　(d) >5,000

25-20. Hardness of aluminium oxide abrasives in KHN is about:
(a) 800–820　　　　　　(b) 1,200–2,000
(c) 2,400–2,600　　　　(d) >5,000

25-21. Diamond particles are bonded to rotary points or discs by:
  (a) Heat resistant polyamide resinoids and Ni electro-plating
  (b) Sintering and hot pressing
  (c) Vitreous ceramics
  (d) None of these

25-22. Precautions while abrading:
  (a) Unidirectional movement away from operator
  (b) Least pressure
  (c) Chose correct abrasives in descending order of particle-sizes
  (d) All of the above

25-23. Polishing refers to:
  (a) Removal of unwanted materials by wearing
  (b) Obtaining Beilby micro-crystalline surface
  (c) Electro-forming
  (d) Wearing by chemicals

25-24. Precautions while polishing:
  (a) Apply adequate pressure
  (b) Multi-directional movement
  (c) Use F, FF or FFF particles in descending order
  (d) All of the above

25-25. Best polishing agent for gold alloys:
  (a) French chalk
  (b) Rouge-Fe_2O_3
  (c) Diamond pastes
  (d) $CaCO_3$, CaH_2PO_4, $NaHCO_3$

25-26. Best polishing agent for PBM alloys:
  (a) French chalk
  (b) Rouge-Fe_2O_3
  (c) Diamond pastes
  (d) $CaCO_3$, CaH_2PO_4, $NaHCO_3$

25-27. Best polishing agent for heat-cure acrylic-dentures:
  (a) French chalk
  (b) Rouge-Fe_2O_3
  (c) Pumice
  (d) $CaCO_3$, CaH_2PO_4, $NaHCO_3$

25-28. Best polishing agent in dentifrices:
(a) Pumice
(b) Rouge-Fe_2O_3
(c) Diamond pastes
(d) $CaCO_3$, CaH_2PO_4, $NaHCO_3$

25-29. Glazing technique is used for finishing:
(a) Ceramics
(b) PBM alloy RPDs
(c) Silver amalgam
(d) Tri-cure glass ionomer cements

25-30. Glaze composite resin is applied for finishing:
(a) Micro-filled composite resins
(b) Cast-glass-ceramics
(c) Large particle-composites
(d) Compomers

25-31. Fine powders of $ZrSiO_2$, ZnO, SnO are used for polishing:
(a) Noble metal alloy castings   (b) Acrylics
(c) 18–8 stainless steel   (d) ICZ incerams

25-32. Dentifrices are used regularly for removing:
(a) Food debris   (b) Stains, pellicles
(c) Microorganisms   (d) All of the above

25-33. Sorbitol or glycerines are used in dentifrices as:
(a) Detergents   (b) Humectants
(c) Binders   (d) Desensitizers

25-34. Potassium nitrate or strontium chlorides are used in dentifrices as:
(a) Detergents   (b) Humectants
(c) Binders   (d) Desensitizers

25-35. Sodium lauryl sulphate is used in dentifrices as:
(a) Detergent   (b) Humectant
(c) Binder   (d) Desensitizer

25-36. Abrasives used in dentifrices are:
(a) Lavigated alumina   (b) Zirconium oxide
(c) $CaCO_3$, $NaHCO_3$ (d) Pumice

25-37. Disodium, tetra-sodium or potassium pyrophosphates are used in dentifrices as:
  (a) Desensitizers   (b) Humectants
  (c) Detergents   (d) Tarter controllers

25-38. Factors effecting abrasivity of dentifrices:
  (a) Hardness, size, content of abrasives
  (b) Intraoral factors
  (c) Nature of brushes and frequency of brushing
  (d) All of the above

25-39. Abrasives used in prophy-pastes are:
  (a) Lavigated alumina, zirconium silicate
  (b) French-chalk
  (c) $NaHCO_3$
  (d) CaH_2PO_4

25-40. Prophy-pastes are used for removing:
  (a) Hard calculus-deposits   (b) Stains, pellicles
  (c) Both   (d) None

25-41. Air-abrasion technique with alumina or zirconia particles of sizes 25–30 microns (μm) is used for:
  (a) Finishing acrylic dentures
  (b) Polishing ceramics
  (c) Polishing compomers
  (d) Remove hard deposits and stains on tooth surface

Answers to Multiple Choice Questions Chapterwise

Chapter 1. Orientation to dental sciences

1	a	2	b	3	c	4	d	5	d
6	(a-5, b-7, c-6, d-3)	7	c	8	d	9	d		

Chapter 2. Properties of dental materials and some solved numerical problems

1	b	2	d	3	c	4	d	5	d
6	a	7	a	8	d	9	a	10	c
11	d	12	a	13	d	14	a	15	b
16	c	17	c	18	c	19	d	20	b
21	(a-3, b-8, c-2, d-6, e-4)			22	(a-8, b-2, c-1, d-3, e-7, f-5)				
23	c	24	d	25	d	26	a		
27	d	28	(a-1, b-2, c-5, d-7, e-8)			29	b		
30	b	31	a	32	a	33	d	34	c
35	b	36	c	37	d	38	b	39	a
40	d	41	a	42	c	43	d	44	c

Chapter 3. Impression materials

1	d	2	d	3	d	4	a	5	d
6	d	7	a	8	c	9	a	10	b
11	d	12	a	13	a	14	a	15	d
16	a	17	d	18	b	18A	d	19	d
20	d	21	b	22	b	23	d	24	c
25	b	26	a	27	a	28	a	29	b
30	a	31	d	32	b	33	d	34	a

35	d	36	d	37	d	38	c	39	b
40	a	41	c	42	d	43	a	44	b
45	d	46	c	47	d	48	d	49	b
50	a	51	c	52	d	53	d	54	b
55	d								

Chapter 4. Gypsum products (auxiliary materials)

1	d	2	d	3	d	4	b	5	a
6	b	7	c	8	a	9	d	10	c
11	a	12	d	13	a	14	b	15	a
16	d	17	b	18	d	19	c		

Chapter 5. Dental polymer resins

1	d	2	a	3	d	4	d	5	e
6	d	7	a	8	a	9	d	10	d
11	b	12	c	13	c					

Chapter 6. Prosthetic applications of polymer resins

1	d	2	c	3	b	4	c	5	a
6	c	7	a	8	d	9	b	10	d
11	a	12	b	13	a	13a	c	14	b
15	c	16	d	17	b	18	c	19	a
20	b	21	d	22	a	23	b	24	c
25	a	26	d	27	d	28	a	29	c
30	a	31	b	32	d	33	d	34	b
35	d	36	d	37	a	38	d	39	d
40	d	41	d	42	d	43	d	44	a
45	d	46	b	47	a	48	b	49	a
50	c	51	d	52	a	53	d	54	b
55	c	56	b	57	c	58	b	59	a
60	d								

Chapter 7. Biocompatible aspects of dental materials

1	b	2	c	3	a	4	b	5	d
6	c	7	d	8	a	9	a	10	a
11	a								

Chapter 8. Restorative dental materials-cements

1	b	2	c	3	a	4	a	5	c
6	c	7	a	8	d	9	d	10	a
11	b	12	c	13	d	14	d	15	b
16	d	17	c	18	b	19	d	20	a
21	c	22	c	23	d	24	d	25	d
26	b	27	b	28	c	29	c	30	c
31	d	32	d	33	b	34	b	35	c
36	b	37	d	38	d	39	a	40	b
41	b	42	c	43	c	44	b	45	b
46	b	47	a	48	b	49	c	50	b
51	d	52	d	53	d	54	all	55	all
56	d	57	d	58	b	59	a	60	c
61	a	62	b	63	b	64	d	65	b
66	c	67	d	68	b	69	d	70	b
71	d	72	d	73	c	74	b	75	all
76	all	77	c	78	d	79	b	80	c
81	b	82	a	83	d	84	d	85	d
86	d	87	d	88	b	89	d	90	a
91	d	92	a	93	b	94	c	95	d
96	Table 8.1								

Chapter 9. Composite restorative resins

1	a	2	d	3	d	4	c	5	c
6	d	7	c	8	d	9	d	10	b
11	b	12	b	13	a	14	b	15	b
16	c	17	c	18	c	19	a	20	c
21	b	22	b	23	b	24	d	25	c
26	d	27	d	28	d	29	d	30	d
31	b	32	a						

Chapter 10. Bonding of restorations

1	b	2	d	3	b	4	c	5	d
6	b	7	b	8	b	9	d	10	a
11	d	12	b	13	d	14	c	15	b
16	d								

Chapter 11. Direct filling gold

1	b	2	d	3	b	4	c	5	a
6	d	7	d	8	b	9	d	10	c
11	b	12	d	13	d	14	c	15	b
16	b								

Chapter 12. Silver amalgam restorative materials

1	c	2	c	3	d	4	d	5	b
6	c	7	c	8	b	9	d	10	d
11	d	12	a	13	d	14	c	15	a
16	d	17	d	18	d	19	a	20	a
21	d	22	d	23	d	24	c	25	b
26	a	27	a	28	b	29	b	30	c
31	b	32	d	33	a	34	b	35	d
36	a	37	d	38	d	39	b	40	d
41	d	42	a	43	d	44	d	45	d
46	b	47	d	48	d	49	d	50	a
51	b	52	c	53	a					

Chapter 13. Dental ceramics

1	b	2	a	3	b	4	c	5	b
6	b	7	d	8	d	9	d	10	a
11	b	12	a	13	c	14	a	15	b
16	c	17	c	18	d	19	a	20	d
21	c	22	a	23	d	24	a	25	b
26	d	27	d	28	d	29	c	30	d
31	a	32	d	33	a	34	d	35	b
36	c	37	a	38	a	39	c	40	b

41	d	42	d	43	a	44	d	45	d
46	a	47	a	48	b	49	a	50	d
51	c	52	d	53	b	54	d	55	a
56	d	57 Table 1.13.1							

Chapter 14. Dental waxes (auxiliary materials)

1	d	2	a	3	c	4	d	5	a
6	d	7	a	8	c	9	b	10	d
11	d	12	d	13	d	14	b		

Chapter 15. Casting investments (auxiliary materials)

1	d	2	a	3	c	4	c	5	b
6	c	7	c	8	c	9	a	10	b
11	a	12	d	13	a	14	d	15	d
16	a	17	a	18	b	19	b	20	d
21	a	22	c						

Chapter 16. Solidifications of metals and alloys (metallurgy)

1	d	2	b	3	d	4	a	5	a
6	c	7	d	8	d	9	d	10	b
11	c	12	d	13	d	14	c	15	b
16	b	17	c	18	b	19	b	20	a
21	a	22	b	23	b	24	d	25	b
26	c	27	a	28	b	29	d	30	d
31	d								

Chapter 17. Dental casting alloys

1	b	2	c	3	a	4	b	5	a
6	a	7	a	8	b	9	d	10	d
11	d	12	b	13	c	14	d	15	b
16	d	17	d	18	d	19	d	20	b
21	c	22	d	23	b	24	a	25	c
26	b	27	d	28	b	29	b	30	d

31	a	32	c	33	a	34	d	35	d
36	d	37	b	38	c	39	a	40	a
41	a	42	d.	43	d. Tables 17.1 to 17.5				

Chapter 18. Casting procedurs and casting defects

1	a	2	a	3	a	4	b	5	b
6	a	7	a	8	b	9	d	10	d
11	c	12	b	13	b	14	d	15	d
16	c	17	a	18	b	19	c	20	d
21	a	22	b	23	a	24	b	25	d
26	a	27	d	28	b	29	b	30	b
31	a	32	c	33	d	34	a	35	b
36	a	37	d	38	d	39	a		

Chapter 19. Wrought alloys

1	d	2	b	3	d	4	d	5	a
6	c	7	a	8	d	9	c	10	c
11	a								

Chapter 20. Carbon-steels and stainless steels

1	a	2	d	3	a	4	d	5	c
6	a	7	c	8	a	9	b	10	c
11	b	12	a	13	d	14	a	15	c

Chapter 21. Materials used in orthodontia

1	d	2	d	3	c	4	a	5	c
6	c	7	d	8	d	9	a	10	a
11	a	12	a	13	a	14	b	15	d
16	d	17	a	18	d	19	a	20	a
21	d	22	a	23	b	24	d	25	d

Chapter 22. Brazing—soldering and welding

1	a	2	d	3	d	4	d	5	b
6	a	7	d	8	a	9	c	10	a
11	c	12	a	13	c	14	d	15	a
16	c	17	a	18	b	19	d	20	c
21	c	22	***						

Chapter 23. Tarnish and corrosion

1	d	2	d	3	d	4	d	5	b
6	d	7	c	8	c	9	b	10	d
11	All								

Chapter 24. Dental implants

1	a	2	c	3	a	4	a	5	c
6	d	7	a	8	c	9	b	10	a
11	d	12	d	13	a	14	c		

Chapter 25. Cutting abrasion and finishing mechanisms and tools

1	d	2	a	3	b	4	d	5	d
6	b	7	c	8	a	9	a	10	b
11	d	12	c	13	b	14	a	15	d
16	d	17	d	18	a	19	c	20	b
21	a	22	d	23	b	24	d	25	b
26	c	27	a	28	d	29	a	30	c
31	c	32	d	33	b	34	d	35	a
36	c	37	d	38	d	39	a	40	c
41	d								

Theory–Viva Voce and Spotters

Introduction

Spotter-test is one of the methods used in the university examinations, to assess the detailed knowledge of the properties and clinical applications of the materials used in dental sciences. Usually about fifteen or twenty samples of dental materials are arranged. Students have to write, the exact identifications, detailed compositions, a few (biological, mechanical and thermal) properties, applications, advantages and disadvantages, briefly, in three or four minutes time.

Color plates: For all spotters materials, with same reference numbers are provided in section D, to help identification and remembering.

Viva voce or oral test is conducted during the dental materials practical examination time, in detail, to assess the real in-depth knowledge of the candidate, and the awards are added to the written theory examinations.

The authors have explained the expected method of answering the usually asked *viva voce as well as spotter questions,* very briefly, in view of *theory* and *viva voce* examinations. These brief answers will definitely help them to analyze and remember the salient features of the materials used in dentistry and to answer theory as well as viva voce examinations.

1. Gypsum Products
(Cast and Die—Auxiliary Materials)

1. Gypsum products, $CaSO_4.\frac{1}{2}H_2O$ of different types (1, 2, 3, 4, 5), are obtained from gypsum ore, $CaSO_4.2H_2O$ by dry and wet calcinations.

Type I gypsum product—impression plaster—β calcium sulphate hemihydrate—$CaSO_4 \cdot \frac{1}{2}H_2O$ dispensed as powder (now out-dated).

Composition, setting reaction, setting time, properties, etc., *refer* to Table 2.1.1.

Uses: Impression plaster is rigid and non-elastic. Earlier used as secondary wash impression for edentulous cases without severe undercuts. Also can be used for partially edentulous case with one or a few teeth, or edentulous case with severe undercuts with special techniques using soluble plaster.

2. Type II gypsum product—dental/model plaster β calcium sulphate hemihydrate—$CaSO_4 \cdot \frac{1}{2}H_2O$ dispensed as powder. For composition, setting action, properties, etc., *refer* to Table 2.1.1.

Uses: To prepare edentulous models for acrylic dentures fabrication procedures, for articulation procedure, flasking wax denture (three pour techniques), base for the stone cast.

3. Type III gypsum product—wet calcined, autoclaved dental stone: Hydrocal—class I stone—$\alpha\text{-}CaSO_4 \cdot \frac{1}{2}H_2O$ dispensed as powder.

Composition, setting reaction, setting time, properties, etc., *refer* to Table 2.1.1.

(*Note:* Supplied in many colors—green, yellow, etc.

Surface hardness =60 RHN.

Uses: To prepare dentulous study models for treatment planning in orthodontia, master cast for fabrication procedures, flasking wax denture and binder in gypsum bonded investment material.

4. Type IV gypsum product—high strength die stone—densite—improved stone—class II stone—$\alpha\text{-}CaSO_4 \cdot \frac{1}{2}H_2O$ dispensed as powder.

Manufacturing method: Prepared by boiling gypsum in 30% $CaCl_2$ or 0.5% sodium succinate solution and added with small amounts of uncalcined gypsum, chemical accelerators, retarders, *balancing agent = 4% K_2SO_4 + 0.4% borax*, color.

Table 2.1.1: Comparative properties of gypsum products

Gypsum varieties	Type I	Type II	Type III	Type IV	Type V
Compositions (uncalcined gypsum and anhydrite, accl (K_2SO_4), ret (Borax) are common to all types)	β HH (same as type II), added with balancing agent (4% K_2SO_4 + 0.4% borax to decrease setting expansion only), sugar or potato starch to form soluble plaster, alizarin S as a coloring material	β HH	α HH, balanced	α HH, balanced	α HH, acc + ret + surfactant (lignin sulfonate)
Crystals	Spongy, irregular	Spongy, irregular	Prismatic, regular	Fine, prismatic, regular	Fine, prismatic, regular
Water/powder (min = 18.6)%	55–75 approximate	40–55	28–35	22–28	19–22
Vicat ST (min) (ADA)	3–5	8–16	8–16	8–16	8–16
NSE (max) % (ADA)	<0.15%, minimized by adding balancing agents	0.3	0.2	0.1, (lowest)	0.1–0.3
Wet, 1-hr comp strength (MPa) (ADA)	Very low	>8.5	>27.5	>34.5	>48
Dry compressive strength (MPa)	10–15	30–50	60–70	70–90	>80
Setting action, reactions of all gypsum products	Solubilities HH = 0.8% and DH 0.2%—supersaturation—form nuclei of crystallization—spherulites-grow—intermesh: $2CaSO_4.\frac{1}{2}H_2O + 3H_2O \rightarrow 2CaSO_4.2H_2O$ + heat (3,900 cal/gm mol)				

For **composition, setting reaction, properties, etc.** *refer* to Table 2.1.1.

Surface hardness = 80 RHN.

Viva voce and practical spotters 147

Uses: Used to prepare hard dies in the fabrications procedures of *noble metal alloy* appliances by lost wax casting technique.

5. Type V gypsum product—high strength and high expansion die stone—α-CaSO₄½H₂O, dispensed as powder.

Manufacturing method: Prepared by boiling gypsum in 30% calcium chloride or 0.5% sodium succinate solution and added with small amounts of uncalcined gypsum, chemical accelerators, retarders, *surfactants like lignin sulfonate,* to improve wetting.

For composition, setting action, properties, etc. *(refer* to Table 2.1.1).

Uses: Used to prepare hard and *enlarged dies* in the fabrications procedures of *predominantly base metal (PBM)* alloy appliances by lost wax casting technique, for compensating larger casting shrinkage.

6. Smaller and bigger Gilmore needles (GN)

Tip diameters: Smaller = $^1/_{12}$" and bigger—$^1/_{24}$"

Weights: Smaller ¼ lb and bigger 1 lb

Uses: Smaller GN for measuring initial setting time and bigger GN for final setting times (ST) of gypsum products.

Factors to increase ST: Higher, W/P, retarders and shorter mixing time.

Factors to decrease ST: Lower W/P, more accelerators and uncalcined gypsum, finer particles, speed or longer mixing time and fresh stock.

The terms used

Gloss disappearance time: It is the time interval from the instant of addition of powder to water, until the surface gloss of excess water, just disappears.

Initial setting time: It is the time interval from the instant of addition of powder to water, until the smaller GN of weight ¼ lb and tip diameter 1/12" just fails to produce indentation.

Final setting time: It is the time interval from the instant of addition of powder to water, until the bigger GN of weight 1 lb and tip diameter 1/24" just fails to produce indentation.

7. Vicat penetrometer

Load: 300 gm and needle diameter = 1 mm.

Vicat's standard ST: This is the time interval from the instant of addition of powder to water, until this Vicat needle fails to penetrate a depth of 5 cm in GP mix.

Vicat ADA standard ST for GP, type I, = 3–5 min ther types, = 8–16 minutes.

Factors affecting ST: *Same as for spotter 1.*

Diagrams: Ref 1.

2. Impression Materials (Auxiliary Materials)

Impression materials are used to record exact accurate negative replica of the oral structure, with all finer details, without any dimensional changes.

8. Impression trays

9. Type I low fusing impression compound (Table 2.2.1).

Table 2.2.1: Composition of impression compound		
Compositions	*Wt%*	*Functions*
Natural or synthetic resins-Copal resin	20%	Thermoplasticity and gives qualities of flow and cohesions
Rosin	20%	Strength
Waxes (beeswax, carnauba wax or paraffin wax	7%	Thermoplasticity produces smooth surface
Various types of oils and fats (stearic acid, palmitic acid, shellac, gutta-percha)	3%	Plasticizer to improve the flow, plasticity workability and hardens the compound
French chalk, talc, diatomaceous earth	50%	Fillers to improve the strength and to reduce thermal contraction
Rouge (Fe_2O_3) ferric oxide	Trace	Color contrast

Mucocompressive, thermoplastic, nonelastic impression material—dispensed as cake form of about 6 mm thickness.

Flow: At 37°C <6% and at 45°C >85% (when a cylindrical disc of 10 mm diameter. 6 mm height held under 2.5 kg load for 10 min).

Disadvantages

- Nonelastic and should be used only for edentulous cases.
- Mucocompressive—poor flow and does not reproduce finer surface details required.
- Large COTE (300–500 ppm/°C), and poor conductor of heat, which leads to distortion by internal stress relaxation.

Uses: For preliminary impression of edentulous arches, for complete dentures.

10. Type I greenstick compound: Low fusing compound for tracing or border molding, dispensed as cone or cylindrical rods of about 10 cm length and 6 mm in diameter and green in color.

Impression technique: Dry kneading technique, i.e. warming over a gas flame.

Flow: At 37°C <6% and at 45°C >85%

Fusion temp: 43°–45°C

Uses

- For border molding technique to record functional depth of sulcus.
- Copper tube impression technique in combination with light body elastomers.

11. Type II impression compound—tray compound

Composition: Thermoplastic resins, waxes, fillers and color pigments.

Flow at 37°C and 45°C: < 2% and 70–85% respectively.

Fusion temp: >70°C

Uses: Fabrication of special trays for recording secondary impressions.

Disadvantages: Lacks strength and is dimensionally unstable. Hence, cold cure acrylic resin is now used.

Note: Type II tray compound is now outdated. At present shellac base plate sheet, made up of thermoplastic material and self cure acrylic is used for special trays and record base fabrications.

12. Zinc oxide eugenol impression pastes: Mucostatic, inelastic, chemically setting, corrective wash impression material—dispensed as base and reactor pastes.

Setting reaction (SR): When equal lengths of two pastes are mixed, in presence of moist air.

Table 2.2.2: Compositions

Ingredients of base paste	Wt%	Functions
Zinc oxide	87	Reactive ingredients
Fixed vegetable or mineral oils	13	Paste former, plasticizer, retarders, masks eugenol irritations
CaCl$_2$ (sometimes)	2	Accelerator

Ingredients of reactor paste	Wt%	Functions
Oil of cloves or eugenol	12	Reactive ingredients
CaCl$_2$ or MgCl$_2$	5	Accelerator
Gum or polymerized resin	50	Facilitates the speed of the reaction and smoother, homogeneous mix
Fillers (silica, kaolin, talc)	20	Paste former, increases strength
Lanolin	3	Plasticizer
Resinous balsam (Canada or pure balsam)	10	Increases flow and facilitates mixing
Color pigments		Trace—homogeneous mixing indicators

$$ZnO + H_2O \rightarrow Zn(OH)_2$$
$$Zn(OH)_2 (Base) + 2HE (Acid) \rightarrow ZnE_2 + 2H_2O$$
Zinc oxide eugenolate (chelate product)

- *The water (moisture) byproduct causes autocatalytic reaction*

Acceleraters: Moisture, $CaCl_2$, $MgCl_2$, glacial acetic acid, primary alcohols, etc.

Retarders: Vegetable (linseed) or mineral oils, mixing at lower temp (not below dew point).

Table 2.2.3: Properties of type I and type II ZnOE impression materials

Types	Consistencies: 500 g load for 10 min—disc diameter	Setting times		Hardness (Krebs penetrometer depth)
		Initial	*Final*	
I. Hard set: Thinner and fast setting	30–50 mm	3–6 min	<10 min	<0.5 mm
II. Soft set: Thicker and slow setting	20–45 mm	3–6 min	<15 min	0.8–1.5 mm

Uses: For secondary or corrective wash impressions of edentulous arches in special trays for fabrication steps of complete dentures.

Advantages

- Mucostatic—gives accurate reproduction of finer details
- Dimensionally stable.
- Can be added to and readapted if found faulty (*corrective wash impression*).
- Adhere well to the surfaces of shellac bases or resin trays (no tray adhesive is required).

Disadvantages

- Nonelastic—cannot be used for severe undercuts, or dentulous cases.
- Some patients feel unpleasant, burning sensation, irritant, and allergic.

Modifications

- *Surgical pastes:* Intraoral bandage after surgical procedures in the mouth. It has more fillers, more plasticizers and eugenol.

- *Bite registration pastes*: To record the occlusal relationship. It has petroleum jelly as plasticizer.
- *Non-eugenol pastes:* For secondary impressions in patients, allergic to eugenol.

13. Non-eugenol impression pastes: Ortho-ethoxybenzoic acid—mucostatic, inelastic, chemically setting—corrective wash impression material—dispensed as base (ZnO) and reactor pastes (EBA).

Compositions: *Refer to Table 2.2.2 (ZnOE)—only eugenol is replaced by ortho-ethoxybenzoic acid*

Setting reaction: *When equal lengths of two pastes are mixed together* [base paste—ZnO and reactor paste—ortho-ethoxybenzoic acid (EBA)]

$$ZnO + 2RCOOH \rightarrow (RCOO)_2 Zn + H_2O$$

Advantages: Non-irritant, and others same as for ZnOE pastes.

14. Agar-agar reversible hydrocolloid gel: Mucostatic-elastic impression/duplicating material—dispensed as gel in sealed container, for duplicating, or disposable syringes for impressions.

Table 2.2.4: Composition of agar-agar gel		
Ingredients	*Wt%*	*Functions*
Agar	13–17	Dispersed phase of sol, form fibrils, brush-heap structures of gel
Borax	0.2–0.5	Modifier; to improve the viscosity of the sol and strength of the gel
Potassium sulphate	1–2	Gypsum surface hardener
Alkyl benzoate	0.1	Preservative
Diatomaceous earth	0.3–0.5	Fillers
Water	85	Dispersal continuous phase in the sol
Thymol	Trace	Bactericide
Glycerin	Trace	Plasticizer
Color and flavoring agent	Trace	For appearance and acceptability

Steps of gelation: On cooling below 40°C

Sol → fibrils (micelles) → brush heaps → gel by intermeshing of brush heaps

Gel → sol on heating above 70°C.

Sol → gel below 38°C. This temperature lag is hysteresis.

Impression techniques

Normal technique

- Gel is liquefied at 100°C, stored at 65°C and just before using, tempered at 46°C for 10 mins to control flow in the tray.
- Then the sol from cartridge is injected over the prepared tooth, the more viscous sol is carried in special tray and held in contact, until gelation completes. *Dislodge with a single sudden jerk (?)*

Wet field technique

- The prepared tooth surface is flooded by hot water. Then agar-agar syringe material is quickly injected to cover the occlusal and incisal areas. Immediately agar-agar tray material is held in contact with this, so that gelation and bonding of two take place simultaneously.

Laminate technique

- The agar-syringe material is injected into the prepared cavity areas and the chilled alginate mix in the tray is held firmly in contact. Agar gelates soon by the *contact of chilled alginate.*

Properties of agar-agar

- Low compression strength = 0.5 to 0.6 MPa.
- Low tear strength = 400–600 gm/cm.
- Poor elastic recovery = 98.5% and poor dimensional stability due to *syneresis* (contraction due to the exudation of fluids) and *imbibitions* (swelling by absorption of water).

Factors to increase gel strength

- Greater concentration of dispersed phase and modifier borax in the sol
- Lower temperature

- Controlled by manufacturer by fillers
- **Rate of loading**—faster the loading of *viscoelastic material*, greater are the resistance to deformation, tear strength and elastic recoveries. Hence, the impression should be *dislodged with a single sudden jerk.*

Characteristic properties of gels

- **Syneresis:** *Shrinkage* due to loss of water or fluid by exudation.
- **Imbibition:** *Swelling or expansion* by absorption of water/fluids, lost earlier
- **Hysteresis: Lag or difference** between the liquefaction (sol formation) and gelation temperatures (for agar-agar 70°C and 40°C) is known as hysteresis.
- **Effect of rate of loading:** Faster loading, greater mechanical properties, and greater elastic recoveries.

Failures: Grainy surface, separation of syringe and tray materials, tearing, external bubbles, irregular voids, distortions, rough and chalky cast surface—causes and remedies.

15. Irreversible hydrocolloid alginate—elastic, mucocompressive impression material dispensed as powder.

Table 2.2.5: Composition of alginate powder		
Ingredients	*Wt%*	*Functions*
Soluble salts of Na, K, or NH$_4$ alginates	15	Forms sol in water and gelates
Calcium sulphate dihydrate	15–16	Reacts and cause gelation by cross-linking
Tri-sodium phosphate	2–3	Retarder (delays gelation, increases or controls the working time)
Diatomaceous earth	50–60	Fillers, gives body, increases strength
Zinc oxide	4	Fillers
Potassium titanium fluoride	3	Gypsum surface hardener, smooth glossy surface
Flavoring agent (winter green or peppermint)	Trace	More acceptable to the patient

Steps of gelation

On mixing powder with water (W/P = 2.5:1 by volume or 24 ml/scoop)

- $2Na_3PO_4 + 3CaSO_4 \rightarrow Ca_3(PO_4)_2 + 3Na_2SO_4$, until all $CaSO_4$ is exhausted. This delays gelation and provides working time.
- Na_n Alginate + n/2 $CaSO_4$ → Ca n/2 Alginate + n/2 Na_2SO_4 (gelation)

Factors effecting gel strength

- Decrease in W/P ratio within limits, increases strength.
- Both under-and overspatulation decreases strength.
- Inhomogeneous mixing decreases strength.

Syneresis, imbibition: (*refer* to Table **2.2.6** agar-agar)

Properties

- **Setting time:** Type I: Fast set = 1–2 min
  Type II: Slow (normal) set = 2–4 min
- **Compressive strength (gel strength):** >0.8 MPa
- **Low elastic recovery:** 97%
- **Low tear strength:** 300–700 gm/cm
- **Poor flexibility:** 5–20%

Uses

- For impressions of *dentulous arches* for crowns, bridges and partial dentures.
- As an aqueous irreversible duplicating material to duplicate casts and models in PBM alloy castings.

Failures: Grainy surface, tearing, bubbles, voids, distortions, rough cast surface **(causes and remedies)**

Modifications

- **Chromatic**—color indicating during different stages during manipulation (mixing time and setting time), normal setting/fast setting varieties and dispensed as powder (brand name—Tropicalgin).
- **Dust-free alginates**: Contain de dusting agent—glycerine or glycol to agglomerate the silica particles.
- **Siliconized alginates:** Contain silicon polymer—stronger material, dispensed as tray and syringe consistencies.

- Alginates containing **disinfectants,** like quaternary ammonium salts or chlorohexamine.
- **Alginates of any desired setting times,** hard or soft varieties, etc. are available.

16. Polysulphide: Elastomeric impression material dispensed as base and reactor pastes (thiokol, mercaptan).

Table 2.2.6: Compositions of polysulphids		
Ingredients of base paste	*%*	*Functions*
Moderately—low molecular wt polysulphides prepolymer with terminal SH groups	74–80	Undergoes polymerization, viscosity increases
Moderately—low molecular wt polysulphides prepolymer with pendent SH groups	2	Causes limited cross-linking, forms elastic rubber and reduces permanent deformation
Reinforcing fillers (according to L,M,H,P bodies)	16, 25, 35, 50	Increases strength and controls viscosity
Dibutyl phthalate	0.5	Plasticizer
Ingredients reactor paste	*%*	*Functions*
PbO_2	78	Oxidizing agent causes polymerization and cross-linked by SH group
Sulphur	0.5–3	To facilitate the reaction (promoter)
Dibutyl phthalate and inert oil	Trace	Plasticizer
Deodorants	Trace	Reduces unpleasant smell

Condensation polymerization: When two equal lengths of the two pastes are mixed, condensation polymerization with limited cross-linking and liberation of water (by product) takes place cross-linking to form polysulphide rubber.

$$\text{Polysulphide prepolymer} + PbO_2 \xrightarrow[\text{Catalyst}]{\text{Sulphur}} \text{Polysulphide rubber}$$
(with terminal and
pendent SH group) + H_2O

Flexibility: 14–17% (*highest flexibility in elastomers*)

Tear strength (large) = 2,500–7000 gm/cm.

Elastic recovery = 97%.

Surface hardness: Light body = 20, medium body = 30, heavy body = 45 (which increases with filler contents) as measured with shore A durometer.

Factors effecting dimensional changes

- Polymerization shrinkage during cross-linking.
- Loss of byproducts such as H_2O.
- Large thermal contraction—COTE = 150 ppm/°C.
- Incomplete elastic recovery (as it is *viscoelastic*).

Disadvantages

- Disagreeable *odour* and taste due to the presence of PbO_2
- Dimensional change due to evaporation of byproducts (H_2O)
- Stains clothes
- Slow setting—may cause distortion

17. Condensation polysilicones elastomeric impression material—room temperature vulcanizing (RTV) silicones dispensed as base paste and reactor pastes (or liquid).

Compositions: *Refer* to Table 2.2.7.

Steps of polymerization: Condensation polymerization.

Setting reaction: Moderately low molecular wt silicone pre-polymer with OH terminal group + ethyl silicate → ortho silicate rubber + C_2H_5 (OH)—volatile byproduct.

Flexibility: 4–9% (low)

Elastic recovery (high): 99.5%—very good

High tear strength: 3500 gm/cm—very good

Surface hardness: 43 (regular body)—adequate

Factors effecting dimensional changes (similar to poly-sulphides)

- Polymerization shrinkage about 1% (linear).
- Shrinkage due to liberation of byproduct.
- Large thermal contraction (COTE = 190 ppm/°C).
- Incomplete elastic recovery (as it is *viscoelastic*).

Uses: Impression techniques in elastomers (*refer* to Table 2.2.10).

Table 2.2.7: Compositions of condensation polysilicone	
Ingredients base paste	*Functions*
Moderately low molecular wt polysilicone prepolymer with hydroxyl (OH) terminated group	It undergoes polymerization and cross-linking to form a rubber
Reinforcing fillers (35–75%)	Controls strength and viscosity
Ingredients of reactor paste	*Functions*
Tri- or tetra-functional ethyl silicate	Cross-linking polymerization
Organometallic compound, tin octoate	Catalyst or activator
Reinforcing fillers (colloidal silica)	Controls strength and viscosity
Color pigments	To indicate complete uniform mixing

18. Addition polysilicone: Elastomeric impression material dispensed as base and reactor pastes of light (syringe), regular (medium), heavy and putty consistencies.

Note: Also supplied as pseudoplastic monophase two pastes systems for single mix single impression technique.

Steps of polymerization: Free radical addition polymerization

Setting reaction

Silane terminal siloxane + vinyl terminal siloxane (without byproduct) $\xrightarrow[\text{(catalyst)}]{\text{H}_2\text{PtCl}_6}$ Silicone rubber

Properties

Flexibility: Low = 3%

Elastic recovery: Excellent = 99.93% *(highest in elastomers)*

Tear strength: Good 3500 gm/cm can be used in thin sections.

Hardness: 55 (regular body)—measured by shore A durometer.

Factors effecting dimensional changes

- Large thermal contraction (COTE = 190 ppm/°C)
- Incomplete elastic recovery (as it is viscoelastic)

Table 2.2.8: Compositions of addition polysilicone	
Ingredients of base paste	*Functions*
Polydimethyl hydrogen siloxane (with terminal H)	Reactive ingredients (takes part in polymerization reaction)
Reinforcing fillers: Light = 16%, regular 25%, heavy = 36% and in putty body >50%	Controls the viscosity of the set material and modifies physical properties
Ingredients of reactor paste	*Functions*
Polydimethyl vinyl siloxane	Reactor
Reinforcing fillers (powdered silica)	Increase strength, modifies physical properties
Chloroplatinic acid (H2PtCl6)	Catalyst
Low molecular weight liquid polymer (polydimethyl vinyl siloxane)	Reactor (reduce viscosity)
Finely divided platinum or palladium	Scavenger for H_2 gas
Color pigments	For evaluating complete mixing and identification

- Negligible polymerization shrinkage (1%)
- Dimensional change is mainly due to thermal contraction (COTE 190 ppm/°C)

19. Polyether elastomeric impression material dispensed as 3 paste systems—base, reactor and body modifier (thinner) and available in 3 consistencies: L, R and H

Setting reaction:
Imine terminated polyether + sulphonic acid ester → polyether rubber (no byproduct)

Steps of polymerization: Cationic ring opening addition polymerization via imine end groups.

Flexibility: Low = 2%

Elastic recovery: 98.9%

Table 2.2.9: Compositions of polyether	
Base paste ingredients	*Functions*
Imine terminated polyether of low molecular weight	Undergoes cross-linking to form rubber
Colloidal silica	Fillers
Glycol ether phthalate	Plasticizers
Reactor paste	*Functions*
Ester derivative of aromatic sulphonic acid	Releases cations, opens ring and cause cross-linking
Colloidal silica	Filler
Glycol ether phthalate	Plasticizer
Body modifier	*Functions*
Octyl phthalate (thinner) + 5% methylcellulose	It reduces the stiffness/viscosity of the unset material and gives more working time

Tear strength: 2,700 gm/cm—least, compared to other elastomers.

Hardness = 62—measured by shore A durometer for regular body

Factors effecting dimensional changes

Good dimensional stability is due to

- Addition polymerization, no byproducts
- Less polymerization shrinkage—negligible volumetric contraction = <0.4%
- Larger COTE, 300 ppm/°C
- Polyether is *inherently hydrophilic* in nature. Hence, absorbs water and swells under most clinical condition

Failures: Rough, uneven and chalky surfaces, bubbles, irregular voids, distortions.

20. Impression techniques: Elastomers available in L, R, H, and P consistencies, are used for the following impression techniques (*note putty wash technique not used for polyether*)

Table 2.2.10: Impression techniques used in elastomers with diagrams 20	
Impression techniques	*Combinations of different consistencies*
Double mix, single impression	Light + heavy body
Double mix, double impression (reline or putty wash technique)	Putty + light body or putty + regular body
Single mix, single impression	Regular or heavy body, having pseudoplastic property
Tube impression	Regular body or light body on greenstick impression

(*Note:* Polysulphide and polysilicones are supplied in all consistencies (L, R, H, and P) and used for all impression techniques as mentioned above. But polyether is supplied with L, R and H; hence putty wash technique cannot be used.)

Uses: To record accurate dentulous impressions for preparation of crowns, bridges, inlays, onlays, partial dentures, and edentulous arches in the preparation of complete dentures.

3. Denture Fabrication Materials

21. Methyl methacrylate (MMA) monomer of denture base resins—highly volatile clear liquid stored in *amber-colored* bottle.

Composition (*refer* to Table 2.3.1).

Properties: Specific gravity = 0.945, polymerization shrinkage = 21%, normal melting temperature = –48°C, boiling temperature = 100.8°C., at 1 atmospheric pressure, mol weight = 100

Structural formula: $CH_2 = C (–CH_3)–C (= O)–OCH_3$.

Applications: Used with PMMA powder to form packable dough in fabrication of denture, special trays, orthodontic appliances, denture repair, etc.

22. Transparent clear liquid, water: Specific gravity = 1.000, highest density at 4°C = 1.000 gm/cc, and at 20°C = 0.9998 gm/cc. Normal boiling temperature = 100°C, at 1 atmosphere pressure and mol. wt H_2O = 18.

(*Note:* Liquids boil at higher temp. at higher pressures)
Applications: *Universal—solvent!*

23. Alginate sol separating medium—colored liquid, (tin-foil substitute, cold-mould seal).
SR: When a thin coating is applied on the land area of plaster mold surface, it forms a thin transparent impervious gel-film of calcium alginate.

Table 2.3.1: Compositions

Ingredients	%
Soluble salt of Na/K/NH$_4$ alginate (forms gel film)	2–3
Alcohol (for evaporation)	3
Glycerine (thickener)	7
Preservatives, color	Traces
Water (balance)	85–88

$Na_n Alg + n/2 \ CaSO_4 \rightarrow Ca_{n/2} \ Alg \ (gel \ film) + n/2 \ Na_2SO_4.$

This impervious thin gel film prevents:

- Diffusion of water from wet plaster into the unpolymerized dough which later cause voids, resulting in crazing.
- Diffusion of monomer from the dough into plaster which polymerize and cause, rough surface and adhesion of plaster to acrylic (plaster-free denture).

Precautions

- Perform complete dewaxing
- Apply carefully two or three layers without trapping air
- Do not apply on the exposed teeth surface, as this film prevents the chemical bonding of teeth with denture.

24. Denture base material—heat cure polymethyl methacrylate (PMMA) powder and methyl methacrylate monomer (MMA) liquid, dispensed as powder or *spherical beads,* manufactured by *suspension or bead polymerization technique* and liquid preserved in amber-colored, closed bottle.

Table 2.3.2: Compositions	
Polymer powder	*Monomer liquid*
Fine beads or powder of Polymethyl methacrylate	Methyl methacrylate monomer
Copolymer	Comonomer
Benzoyl peroxide (initiator)	Ethylene glycol dimethacrylate (cross linking agent)
Barium/bismuth oxides (radio-opacifier)	Dibutyl phthalate (plasticizer)
Color pigments (HgS, Fe_2O_3, CdS)	0.006% hydroquinone (inhibitor)
Dyed organic nylon fibres (natural appearance)	

Stages of mixing: Physically 5 distinct stages are observed, during mixing of powder liquids (in 2.5:1 ratio by weight or 3:1 by volume).

Stage I: *Wet sandy stage*—powder gets wetted, no cohesion.

Stage II: *Sticky stage*—liquid dissolves the surface particles of the powder.

Stage III: *Dough stage*—particles dissolve completely, and the mix becomes non sticky homogeneous, soft dough. This is packing stage.

Stage IV: *Elastic—rubbery stage:* Attained after dough stage.

Stage V: *Stiff stage:* Evaporation of monomer, results a *stiff stage*.

The dough forming time is the interval between the instant of mixing and the non-sticky condition is just reached. (ADA specification no. 12 is <40 min.)

Working (or dough) time is the interval, during which dough stage is retained (ADA specification no. 12 is >5 min) = packing interval

Stages of polymerization: *Stages of addition polymerization by free radicals, initiator, activated by heat, chemicals (dimethyl-p-toluidine) or UV light (λ = 350 nm), or visible light (λ = 468 nm).*

- **Initiation or induction**
  Benzoyl peroxide (BPO) $\rightarrow$ 2R*, R* + M $\rightarrow$ RM*, A etc. (M = monomer)
- **Propagation**
  RM* + M $\rightarrow$ RM1-M*, + M, + M, + M, etc. $\rightarrow$ RM$_n$-M* + heat, 12,500 cal/gm.mol.
- **Termination** is by chain transfer and direct coupling.

Properties of heat cure acrylics

- CS = 75, TS = 65, PL = 30 and MOE—2,450 (units—all in MPa).
- SH = 18–20 (KHN), COTE = 80–120 ppm/°C, K = 0.006 cgs units.
- **All mechanical properties (the above values) are about 5 to 10% lower for cold-cured acrylics as DP is lower.**

Applications: Used for complete denture (CD), removable partial denture (RPD), rebasing and relining the old misfitting dentures, acrylic jacket crown and veneering of the metallic crowns and bridges, athletic mouth protectors, etc.

25. Self-cure polymethyl methacrylate (PMMA) powder and methyl methacrylate (MMA) liquid.

Compositions

Powder: Same as heat acrylic, except the smaller sized particles.

Liquid: Same as heat cure acrylic—with chemical activator, **N-N, dimethyl-p-toluidine.**

Note:

- For the stages of mixing and polymerizations, *refer* to spotter no. 24.
- For comparison between heat cure and self cure acrylics ref Q. 2 Question paper Nov 2015 (YU) page 212).
- For self-cured acrylic, all these intervals are much shorter as *polymerization* (*chemical stages*) begins *instantly on mixing* with evolution of heat, 12,500 cal/gm.mol. Hence, number of trial closures is limited to one or two.
- Curing is done for 2 hr. in a pressure chamber.

Disadvantages: All mechanical, esthetic properties and biocompatibility are inferior, and are allergic due to higher residual monomer.

Advantages: Simpler fabrication steps and better fit.

Applications of self cure acrylic resins: For fabrications of special trays, record base, orthodontic removable appliances, denture repairs, relining, resilient liners (which have more plasticizers), temporary crowns, bridges, etc.

26. Denture repair materials: Both heat and cold cure materials used, are dispensed as polymer powder and MMA monomer liquids (*refer* to RGU QP. in page 213).

27. Denture reliners: Both heat and cold cure materials used are dispensed as polymer powder and MMA monomer liquids (compositions and techniques).

28. Denture soft resilient liners: Both heat and cold cure materials used are dispensed as polymer powder and MMA monomer liquids with larger amounts of dibutyl phthalate-plasticizers. Polysilicones, heat-cured (single paste or gel) or chemical cured two paste systems polysilicones are used. Highly plasticized PVC, polyvinyl chloride or polyurethanes are also available.

29. Short-term tissue conditioners: Powder contains PMMA or its higher copolymers. Liquid contains large molecular sized aromatic plasticizers like butyl phthalate, butyl glycolate, or dibutyl phthalates 50 to 80% in alcohol or ethanol. Recently viscous silicone liquid in thin polythene envelope is used.

30. Maxillofacial reconstruction materials

Requirements

- Permanent skin-like texture, color, flexibility, hygienic, etc.

Materials used

(a) Polysilicones both heat and cold cured (RTV—room temp. vulcanizing types) with intrinsic colour pigments-like, dry earth, rayon fibres, oil paints added using expensive rolling milling machines have initially good flexibility, skin like texture but decrease in service. The disadvantages are
   - High curing temp, 180°C, difficult to trim and polish.
   - Inhygenic—seat for *Candida albican* causes denture stomatitis where mild inflammation and redness of the oral mucosa occurs beneath the denture.

(b) Plasticized PMMA.: Disadvantages—Heavy, low resilience-gradually harden.

(c) Plasticized PVC.: Disadvantages—Costly metal mould, plasticizer leach out–harden.

(d) Latex rubber: Disadvantages: Gradually degenerate, allergic to some patients.

(e) Synthetic rubbers: Tripolymer of butyl acrylate, MMA, methyl metha-acrylamides. Disadventage—short life.

(f) Polyurethanes: Disadventage—short life.

4. Restorative Materials and Cements

31. Zinc Oxide Eugenol cements (conventional)—dispensed as zinc oxide powder and eugenol liquid.

Setting reaction: When powder liquids are mixed, in presence of moisture

Table 2.4.1: Compositions		
Powder	*%*	*Functions*
Zinc oxide	69	Reactive ingredients
White rosin	29.3	Reduces the brittleness
Zn stearate	1	Plasticizer
Zn acetate	0.7	Accelerator
Liquid	*%*	*Functions*
Eugenol	85%	Reactor
Olive oil	15%	Plasticizer

$ZnO + H_2O \rightarrow Zn\,(OH)_2$

$Zn(OH)_2(base) + 2HE\,(acid) \rightarrow ZnE_2 + 2H_2O$

Zinc eugenolate (chelate product)

The *water* formed *is utilized* in the further reaction and hence the reaction is termed as *autocatalytic reaction.*

pH in 3 mins: Almost neutral (*Note: ZnOE and its modifications are almost neutral*)

Compressive strength: 3–40 MPa (low)

Tensile strength: 0.3–6 MPa (low)

Uses (Type I to IV)
- Type I   : Temporary cementation
- Type II   : Permanent cementation
- Type III : Temporary restorations
- Type IV : Cavity liners
- Used as pulp capping agents and root canal sealants.

Specialities
- Obtundent (anesthetics), almost neutral.
- **Contraindications** for use with composite resins and polyacrylates, as eugenol is a solvent to resins (softens), glass ionomer cement, as leaching of eugenol can cause discolorations.

32. Resin modified ZnOE (brand name Kalginol/IRM) dispensed as powder liquid.

Table 2.4.2: Compositions

Powder	Wt%	Functions
Zinc oxide	70	Reactive ingredients
Natural or synthetic resins (PMMA)	30	Increases strength

Liquid	%	Functions
Eugenol	85%	Reactor
Acetic acid	15%	Accelerators
Thymol	Small amount	Antimicrobial (cement)

Setting reaction: Same as ZnOE and has higher compressive strength = 55 MPa.

Uses

- Permanent cementation
- Cavity lining agents and base
- Intermediate restorative material (IRM)
- Restoration of deciduous teeth
- Temporary restoration

(*Note:* IRM—intermediate restorative material and as a base)

Intermediate restoration—should last for a few weeks to months

Specialities: Same as ZnOE.

33. Alumina reinforced EBA (ortho-ethoxybenzoic acid) cement—dispensed in powder liquid system

Uses

- Permanent cementations
- Cavity liners and bases
- Intermediate restorations

Table 2.4.3: Compositions		
Powder	*Wt%*	*Functions*
Zinc oxide	60–70	Reactive ingredients
Fused alumina	25–30	Increases strength
Rosin	Balance	Reduces the brittleness
Calcium chloride	1.2%	Accelerator
Liquid	*Wt%*	*Functions*
Eugenol	37.5%	Reactive ingredients
Ortho-ethoxybenzoic acid	62.5%	Increases strength

Setting reaction: $ZnO + 2\ RCOOH \rightarrow (RCOO)_2\ Zn + H_2O$.

Properties: Due to higher P/L (7:1) ratio, this has

- Higher compressive strength = 50 MPa
- Higher tensile strength = 4–7 MPa
- Less irritation

34. Zinc phosphate cements—dispensed as powder liquid system

Mixing: Powder/liquid ratio—type I—luting = 2.8 gm/ml, and type II—base = 4.8 gm/ml.

Add initially two small increments to reduce initial acidity and increase working time, then spatulate larger increments covering large area to dissipates heat, then smaller increments to adjust consistency.

Setting reaction: On mixing powder liquid, containing Al and zinc phosphate buffer:

$ZnO + Al + H_3PO_4 \rightarrow$ Zinc aluminophosphate gel + H_2O + heat (exothermic).

Acidity: pH at 3 minutes = 1.6–3.5 and at 24 hours = 5–6.

Consistency is found by measuring the diameter of the disc formed by 0.5 ml of standard mix, when held in between two glass plates under 125 gm load for 10 min.

Table 2.4.4: Compositions

Powder—prepared by sintering	Wt%	Functions
Zinc oxide	90	Reactive ingredients
Magnesium oxide	8–9	Lowers sintering temperature
Bismuth trioxide Calcium oxide	Small	Imparts smoothness to the freshly mixed cement
Barium oxide	Small	Radio-opacifier
Silicon dioxide	Small	Inert fillers, gives strength and also aids in sintering.

Liquid in closed bottle with dropper	Wt%	Functions
Phosphoric acid	43	Reactive agent
Water	33 ± 5	Controls pH and rate of setting reaction
Aluminium phosphate or zinc phosphate	16	Buffers—stabilizes the pH of zinc phosphate acids
Aluminum	2.5	Forms cohesive zinc aluminum phosphate
Zinc	7	Moderator

Table 2.4.5: Properties

Properties	Type I (luting)	Type II (base)
Compressive strength, ADA spec	80–100 MPa >75 MPa	110–160 MPa >103 MPa
Tensile strength	5.5 MPa	5–14 MPa
MOE (similar to dentin)	14,000 MPa	22,000 MPa
Film thickness	25–30 microns	30–35 microns
Consistency-disc-diam.- Powder/liquid	30–35 mm 2.8 gm/ml	25–30 mm, 4.8 gm/ml

Uses

- Permanent cementations of inlays, crowns, bridges, etc.
- Cementation of orthodontic bands and brackets.
- Thermal insulating base in small cavities (larger dentin thickness).
- Temporary and intermediate restorative material.

Advantages: Adequate strength for cement base and also low film thickness for luting, pseudoplastic.

Disadvantages: No chemical bonding to tooth enamel, opaque and not anticariogenic, acidic, irritant to pulp.

Modifications

- Hydrophosphate water settable zinc phosphate cement has no benefits.
- Fluoride cements (addition of "F" has no much benefit since it does not leach out.
- Germicidal cements: Silver or copper cements, not used now (prepared by incorporating silver or copper salts).
- Zinc silico-phosphate cement (*refer* to spotter no. 36).

35. Silicate cements: Now not used as it is most irritant

Compositions

Powder: This is glass powder containing silica (40%), alumina (30%) and fluorides of Na, K, Ca (23%) and is prepared by *fritting, i.e. quenching the molten mass and powdering.*

Liquid: Contains phosphoric acid, water and buffers in closed bottle with a nozzle.

When the powder liquid are mixed, *hydrated alumino-silicate gel* is formed. Hence, mixing is done by *folding or overlapping technique to prevent damage to gel structure, using plastic spatula covering minimum area.* The restoration is coated with varnish to prevent syneresis and imbibitions of the gel structure before it completely sets.

Setting reaction: *Powder + liquid* $\rightarrow Al^{+++}, Ca^{++}, Na^+, F^- \rightarrow$ *siliceous gel + phosphates and fluoride matrix.*

Properties

- *The first anticariogenic, anterior restorative cement*
- High prolonged acidity = 2.8 pH at 3 minutes and even after one week pH = 5.
- *Most irritant, can cause pulp-death,*
- *High CS:* 200 MPa, surface hardness: 80 KHN, and low TS: 15 MPa (brittle).
- High solubility, maximum in citric acid of pH = 0.4.

Used earlier for cementation of esthetic restoratives and anterior restorations, cementations. Now obsolete.

Specialities

- Translucency similar to that of porcelain and was used for cementation of porcelain restorations.
- *Anticariogenic property*: Fluorides contribute to the *caries inhibition* in the oral environment by two mechanisms.
  1. *Physiochemical mechanism*—hydroxyapatite + F → fluoroapatite (acid resistant).
  2. *Biological mechanism by enzyme inhibition*—fluoride can enter bacterial cell present in the plaque and inhibit the carbohydrate metabolism, thus preventing the production of acid.

36. Zinc silicophosphate cement. Alternate names: filling synthetic porcelain—zinc silicate—now obsolete).

Compositions: Mixtures of powders, as well as liquids of $ZnPO_4$ and silicate cements.

Setting reaction: Both, but predominantly of silicate cements.

Acidity: Intermediate (less irritant than silicate cement)

CS: Intermediate (>168 MPa, 140–170 MPa)

TS: Intermediate (6–7 MPa)

MOE: Intermediate

Solubilities: In saliva (0.1–0.3%) and more in citric acids, etc., which is less than silicate, but more than $ZnPO_4$ cements

Modifications and uses: Type I—luting porcelain crowns and veneers.

Type II—IRM, temporary posterior restorations.

Speciality: Anticariogenic, translucent and strong cement.

37. Zinc polycarboxylate cement (Zn poly C, Zn poly F, high bond) dispensed as powders liquid system—first adhesive cement

Table 2.4.6: Compositions		
Powder	*Wt%*	*Functions*
ZnO	80%	Reactive ingredients
MgO	10%	Decreases calcination temperature
SiO_2 + Al_2O_3	2–8%	Increases strength
Stannous fluoride	4–5%	Improves physical properties
Liquid		35–45% aqueous solution of polyacrylic acid of moderate molecular weight 25,000–50,000 with copolymers of polyacrylic acid such as itaconic acid and tartaric acid, which reduce the high viscosity of polyacrylic acid

Mixing: Divide one scoop powder on the glass-slab into two or three parts, and mix in minimum area with 1 or 2 drops of liquid. (Mix has glossy appearance, use before *cobwebbing*).

Setting reaction: When the powder is mixed with liquid:

ZnO + polyacrylic acid → Zinc polycarboxylate.

Chemical bonding reactions with tooth enamel and dentin

Adhesion to enamel is achieved by *ionic bonding* of:

–COOH—group with Ca^{++} ions of enamel acting as bridges, –OOC–Ca^-(of enamel)–COO–

Adhesion to dentin is by two methods

- *Hydrogen bonds* are formed between the carboxyl groups of the polyacrylic acid and the amino group of the dentin collagen.
- (Mg^{++}) ions diffuse from the cement particles, form cation bridges between the carboxyl groups of the polyacrylic acids and dentin collagen

Properties

Biocompatibility is due to its *mildness or kindness to the pulp* when it is protected by a thin dentin layer.

- **Acidity: pH = 3.5 at 2 minutes and 6.2 at 24 hours.**
- Weak acid and neutralized soon.
- The acid forms protein complexes blocking dentinal tubules.
- Large sized PAA molecules cannot diffuse through dentinal tubules.

Compressive strength: 55–85 MPa (slightly lower than $ZnPO_4$ cement)

MOE: Luting cement = 4–5 GPa and base cement = 5–6 GPa ($< ZnPO_4$ cement)

Esthetics: Opaque.

Uses

- For permanent cementation of metallic crowns, bridges, etc.
- Cementation of orthodontic bands and porcelain restorations.
- As thermal insulating bases.
- As temporary filling materials.

Specialities

- Direct chemical bonding with tooth structure *(adhesive cement)*
- Excellent biocompatibility and kind to the pulp

Modifications

- *Water settable* zinc polycarboxylate cement containing *freeze dried acrylic acid,* dispensed as single component powder, which can be mixed with distilled water. This has no better properties.

38. Glass-ionomer cement type I—luting cement dispensed as powder liquid system. Alternate names—ASPA (alumina-silicate-polyacrylate), vitremer, polyalkeonates, chemfil, ionofill.

Setting reaction: Aluminosilicate glass powder + polyacrylic acid and copolymers → calcium and aluminum polysalt gel + silica gel.

Calcium polysalt gel formed during initial set is highly susceptible to moisture contamination and water sorption.

Table 2.4.7: Compositions		
Powder (fritting method)	Wt%	Functions
Silica	29.0	Increases hardness and translucency
Alumina	16.5	Reacts with polyacrylic acid to give aluminum polyacrylate matrix
Aluminum fluoride	7.0	Flux—reduces fusion temperature, anticariogenic property
Calcium fluoride	34.0	
Sodium fluoride	3.0	Provide anticariogenic property and improves working characteristic
Aluminum phosphate	10	Controls the setting time
Liquid		45–50% aqueous solution of polyacrylic acids, and its copolymer acids like itaconic acid, maleic acid and tricarboxylic acids, with a small amount of tartaric acid which reduces viscosity of the liquid, increase working time and decrease setting time

A protective *coating of varnish or cocoa-butter* is applied to protect the restoration from moisture contamination until aluminum polysalt gel is formed (in about 30 minutes).

Properties

- **Acidity:** pH at 2 minutes is about 1.8 and in 24 hours = 6.0–almost neutral.
- **Compressive strength:** 90–140 MPa (< silicate cement).
- **Tensile strength:** 6–7 MPa (brittle).
- **Modulus of elasticity:** 7–8 GPa
- **Film thickness:** 25–30 microns.

Specialities

GIC has desirable properties of both silicate and zinc polycarboxylate (hybrid) cements.

- Excellent biocompatibility.
- Direct *chemical bonding* to the tooth structure.
- Translucency similar to that of porcelain and hence used for cementation of porcelain restorations.

- *Anticariogenic property:* Fluorides contribute to the *caries inhibition* in the oral environment by two mechanisms.
- *Physiochemical mechanism: Hydroxyapatite + F → fluoroapatite (acid resistant).*
- *Biological mechanism by enzyme inhibition:* Fluoride can enter bacterial cell present in the plaque and inhibit the carbohydrate metabolism, thus preventing the production of acid.
- Favorable bioactive property and used as *bone substitute.*

Classification, uses

Type   I: Luting of metallic crowns, bridges and ceramic restorations, etc.
Type   II: Restorations.
Type   III: Cavity liners.
Type   IV: Pit and fissure sealants.
Type   V: Orthodontic cementations.
Type   VI: Core building.
Type   VII: Vitremer core build.
Type   VIII: Metal modified—ketac silver
Type   IX: Pediatric, gediatric (ART)

39. Glass-ionomer type II—cements—restorative material dispensed as powder with scoop and liquid (with dropper).

Comp, SR, pH at 3 minutes and 24 hours: Nearly same as Type I—*refer* to 38.

Compressive strength: 140–150 MPa (stronger than type I)

Tensile strength: 6.6 MPa

Surface hardness: 40–50 KHN

Modul of elasticity: 8–9 GPa

Film thickness: 30–40 microns.

Uses

- Restoration of class V and III cavities
- Restoration of abraded and cervical eroded areas without any cavity preparations
- Restorations of deciduous teeth
- Repairing defective margins in restorations.

Specialities: *Refer* to Q. 38, type I GIC

Modifications of GIC
- Metal modified—miracle mix (*refer* to Q. 40) and glass-cermet (*refer* to Q. 41)
- Pediatric or gediatric ART, Fuji IX (*refer* to Q. 42)
- Resin modified GIC—resinomer (*refer* to Q. 43)
- Resin modified tricure compomer (*refer* to Q. 44)
- Core build up—vitrimer GIC Fuji. Fuji VII (*refer* to Q. 45)

40. Metal modified glass-ionomer cement-miracle mix dispensed as powder liquid system

Details
- Composition: Spherical amalgam alloy powder is admixed with type II GIC powder and the liquid used was aqueous solution of polyacrylic acid.
- Due to poor adhesion of silver tin alloy particles into the matrix, the properties of miracle mix were far inferior to those of dental amalgam.
- The alloy particles act as fillers and improve the *properties very slightly,* since these do not bond with the GIC powder, i.e. CS = 180–200 MPa, TS = 10 MPa.
- Anticariogenic property and chemical bonding to tooth are not affected.

41. Metal modified glass–ionomer cement–glass cermet (brand—Ketac Silver) (powder liquid system)

Details: Contains glass + metal (silver) powder *sintered together to high density* that can react with active solution of polyacrylic acid and set.

$$\begin{matrix} \text{Glass powder} \\ \text{(ceramic powder)} \end{matrix} + \begin{matrix} \text{metal modifiers} \\ \text{(Au-Ag) metal} \end{matrix} \rightarrow \begin{matrix} \text{cermet cement} \\ \text{(ceramic metal)} \end{matrix}$$

Properties: Similar to GIC type II (*refer* to Q. 38 and Q. 39)

Disadvantages
- Low fracture resistance due to brittleness.
- More opacity, poor aesthetics.
- Lower SH = 40 KHN.

42. GIC—Fuji IX—pediatric or gediatric restorative material: Compositions, properties, etc. are nearly similar to GIC types I or II (*refer* to Q. 38 and Q. 39)

Uses

- These are high viscosity GICs used in *atraumatic restorative therapy (ART)*, which refers to the restoration of tooth with minimum cavity preparation or minimum instrumentation which is *essential for pediatric and gediatric patients*.
- Mostly used as posterior restorative material.

Advantages

- Easily packable and condensable.
- Early moisture sensitivity is reduced.
- Rapid finishing, carving out immediately.
- Improved wear resistance.
- Low solubility in oral fluids.

43. Resin modified GIC—resin-ionomers (resinomers), hybrid-ionomers, dual or tri cure systems or compomer

Dispensing: Powder liquid systems, or single paste tri-cure (light cure) systems.

Compositions

Powder: Contains ion leachable glass with fluorides, resin matrix (BIS-glycidylomethacrylate) + coupling agents (organosilanes) + initiators (light initiators or chemical initiators or both).

Liquid: Aqueous solution of polyacrylic acid with some carboxyl groups, modified methyl methacrylate and HEMA (hydroxyl-ethyl methacrylate), chemical accelerator (dimethyl aminoethyl methacrylate.

Properties

- Anticariogenic, lower compressive strength = 105 MPa, tensile strength = 20 MPa.
- Surface hardness = 40 KHN, and chemical adhesion to the tooth structure.

Drawbacks

- Exhibits shrinkage on setting.
- Biocompatibility is not very good.
- Susceptible to dehydration, absorbs water, produces significant dimensional changes.

Uses

- Liner under composite resins
- Core build up material
- Fissure sealant
- Cement base material
- Cementation of orthodontic bands

44. Compomer-resin modified tri cure GIC

Dispensed in disposable single paste capsule/syringe systems (or rarely powder liquid).

Composition: Non-reactive organic fillers, reactive glass particles with NaF, polyacid modified monomers and photo-activators.

Setting reactions: Initially, chemical cure (polymerization) and slow acid–base reaction of GIC, then by photoinitiation.

Properties and uses—similar to resin modified GIC (*refer* Q. 43).

45. Vitremer—core build up GIC restorative material Fuji VII glass-ionomer cement

Speciality and use

- World's first high fluoride, non-resin containing—auto cure-glass ionomer cement.
- Excellent material for prevention of caries and used for molar restorations in deciduous teeth and used as core build up material.

46. Cavity varnishes

Compositions: Natural gums (copal resin or rosins, synthetic resins-nitrated cellulose) dissolved in organic solvents like acetone, chloroform or ether and sometimes provided separately.

Use: Applied on cavity walls and floor, protects the pulp in case of amalgam and DFG restorations (thermal conduction).

Contraindications: To resin restorations due to softening by these solvents.

47. Cavity liners: Thin suspensions of $Ca(OH)_2$ powder or ZnOE (type IV), or glass ionomers (type-3).

Use: For coating on the cavity floor to protect the pulp from chemical irritation by neutralising the acid-ions diffusing from acidic restorations. $Ca(OH)_2$ also forms reparative secondary dentin (*refer* to Q. 48).

48. Calcium hydroxide cements: Dycal chemical, cured, dispensed as two paste systems. Dycal—VLC single paste system (Dycal).

Table 2.4.8: Composition of two paste system		
Base paste	*%*	*Functions*
Glycol salicylate	40	Reactive ingredients
Calcium tungstate	16	Radio-opacifiers
TiO_2	14	Fillers
Calcium sulphate	30	Provides strength and color
Reactor paste	*%*	*Functions*
$Ca(OH)_2$	50	Reactive ingredients
ZnO	10	Reactive ingredient
Zn stearate	0.5	Strength

Setting reaction: When the two pastes (equal lengths) are mixed together on a glass slab.

Glycol salicylate + $Ca(OH)_2$ → calcium disalicylate (chelate product)

Properties

- Alkaline, pH = 11–12, forms reparative secondary dentin
- Compressive strength—very low 10–27 MPa.

- Tensile strength—very low: <1.5 MPa, fractures if Ag-amalgam or DFG are condensed.
- Good thermal insulator.
- Ideal for pulp protection.

Specialities

- The only *alkaline cement*, forms secondary (reparative) dentin due to its large alkaline pH and re-mineralization action.
- This is good thermal insulator but has low strength, no chemical bonding, no anticariogenic properties.

Use: Chemically cured as sub-base or liners temporary sealing, VLC for pulp capping, non-setting ZnOE for intra-canal medications.

Note: **Dycal and Calcimol (Voco)VLC systems dispensed as single paste system have:** $Ca(OH)_2$, $BaSO_4$, (radio-opacifiers), urethane dimethacrylate or camphorquinone as photo-initiators and accelerators. These **ingredients** are dispensed in 39.5% ethylene toluene sulfonamide.

49. Gutta-percha dispensed as rods or points, naturally occurring polymeric material which is chemically known as *trans-isomer of poly-isoprene*, obtained from latex of tropical rubber trees

On warming it changes from,

α (alpha) GP, 50°C β (beta) GP 56°–62°C γ (gamma) GP
$\longleftrightarrow$ $\longleftrightarrow$

When GP cone is kept in chloroform or eucalyptus oil it forms thin soft layer which helps condensation and are known as *chloropercha or eucapercha.*

Table 2.4.9: Compositions		
Ingredients	*Wt%*	*Functions*
Gutta-percha	20	Forms the matrix
ZnO	60	Fillers improves the strength
Waxes	5–10	Plasticizers
Barium sulphate	Trace	Radio-opacifiers

Dispensing: It is supplied in the form of small narrow cones of various sizes, 15–18 numbers (15 means the tip diameter of gutta-percha $15/100 = 0.15$ mm (and every one mm from the tip there is an increase of 0.02 mm in size) in various colors indicating diameters.

Chemical formula: $CH_2 = CH - C(CH)_3 = CH_2$.

Properties: Inert, dimensionally stable, thermoplastic, thermal insulator and easily be used.

Applications: Gutta-percha is used for *sealing the root canal* by several techniques such as warm up, cold up, injection, semi-dissolved methods (chloropercha, or eucapercha). It is also used as *functional impression material* for cleft palate cases.

50. Mineral trioxide aggregate (MTA)—root canal repair material (powder)

Composition: Tri-calcium silicate, tri-calcium aluminate, tri-calcium oxide, silicate oxide and bismuth oxide.

Manipulation: MTA is supplied in powder form and one scoop of powder is mixed with one drop of distilled water on glass slab for 30 sec until they become homogeneous with wet sand like consistency. The mix is carried to the selected site by amalgam carrier and condensed.

Setting action

Oxides of calcium in MTA + water $\rightarrow$ calcium hydroxide
Ca from $Ca(OH)_2$ + CO_2 (from pulp tissue) $\rightarrow$ calcite crystals

Setting times: 15 minutes to 3 hours (slow setting)

Compressive strengths: About 65 MPa in 21 days.

Advantages

- Excellent marginal sealing, prevents bacterial migration and penetration of tissue fluids through root canals.
- Prompts the formation of dentin bridge when used in pulp capping.
- Lower solubility than calcium hydroxide and better physical properties.
- Indicated when moisture control is adequate.

Uses

- Reverse root filling (retrograde filling)
- Pulp capping
- Pulpotomy in teeth with incomplete root development
- Internal resorption
- Sealing perforations of root canal

51. RC-Prep (Brand name): Root canal preparation cream supplied in jar or syringes.

Compositions: Urea peroxide (10%) and EDTA (ethylene-diaminetetra-acetic acid—15%) in a special water-soluble base.

Uses

- When RC-Prep reacts with sodium hypochlorite solution, pulp debris is lifted out of the canal. The pulp chamber is brightened, helping to locate additional canals.
- RC-Prep is routinely used for the chemo-mechanical preparation of root canals.
- Helps to remove calcification and also lubricates of the canal to permit more efficient instrumentation.

5. Composite Restorative Resins

52. Composite resins are three-dimensional structures of two or more chemically different, insoluble in each other, materials with another interfacial material (coupling or keying agent) which increases mechanical properties, dimensional stability, and acts as stress absorber

Classifications according to

- **Resin matrix** (Bowen's resin—BisGMA, Bis GMA without OH groups, triethylene glycol dimethacrylate—TEGDMA, etc.
- **Inorganic fillers:** Pyrolytic-precipitated-colloidal glass particles of size distributions, large = 1–50 μm, smal 1–12 μm, micro = 0.04–0.06 μm, **nano <0.01 μm (10 nm)**, hybrids of these, organic resin fillers.
- **Initiators:** Benzoil peroxide (for chemical curing), benzoin methyl ether (for UV), camphorquinone-diketones with

tertiary amines—dimethyl paratoluidine as accelerator (for VLC).

- **Activators:** Chemical-N-N-dimethyl paratoluidine, ultraviolet light of $\lambda = 350$ nm, visible light of = 468 nm or 460–480 nm.
- **Dispensing methods:** Powder-liquids, two pastes, single paste system, disposable capsules.
- **Clinical applications:** Anterior, posterior, core build-up, pit and fissure sealants, prosthodontic veneers, glazes, bonding agents, etc.

53. Compositions of composite resins

1. Organic resin phase—matrix—BisGMA bisphenol glycidyl dimethacrylate with or without—OH—groups, TEGDMA, etc.
2. Inorganic filler (quartz, Al-glass) and organic filler particles (treated with resin and coupling gent) dispersed in resin matrix to increase strength, hardness, transparency, and decrease polymerization shrinkage, COTE, etc.
3. Interfacial phase *coupling or keying agent, vinyl silane or gamma methacryloxy propyl trimethoxy silane,* which combines the filler and resin matrix by chemical bonding. This increases strength, acts like stress absorber, decreases polymerization shrinkage, and COTE.
4. Color pigments (TiO_2, Al_2O_3 BaO, etc., metal oxides).

SR: Composite resins set by highly cross-linked additional polymerization reaction—through chemical or light activation

Bis-GMA + TEGDMA + Initiators + coupling agent coated inorganic fillers $\rightarrow$ Highly cross-linked polymer matrix composite with fillers

Activators and initiators

- For hemical activation initiator is N-N dimethyl para toloudine.
- For U-V light (360 nm) activation initiator is benzoin methyl ether.
- For visible light (460–475 nm) activation initiator is camphorquinone and tertiary amine—dimethyl aminoethyl methacrylate (accelerators).

Light sources

- Light emitting diodes (LED lamps).
- Quartz-Tungsten Halogen (QTH) lamps.
- Plasma Arc Curing (PAC) lamps.
- Argon laser lamps.

Direction of polymerization shrinkage

- Chemically cured composite—*towards centre* of cavity
- VLC—*external surface* of restoration, closest to the light source

Degree of polymerization (conversion)

- Uniform in chemical cure
- Not uniform in VLC, DP is less, away from the light source.

Properties: Depend upon the filler contents, particle size distributions, degree of conversion, etc.

- **CS:** 300–380 MPa
- **TS:** 45–70 MPa
- **COTE:** 25–35 ppm/°C
- **MOE:** 5,000–13,000 MPa
- **SH:** 25–50 KHN.

Advantages over unfilled acrylics

- Superior aesthetics
- Dentists' command set property for UV and VLC composites
- Improved mechanical properties and better wear resistance
- Reduced polymerization and thermal shrinkages
- Higher strength and abrasive resistance for hybrid composites

Disadvantages

- No chemical bonding to tooth, or anticariogenic properties
- The formaldehyde found in VLC, may cause **lichenoide lesions,**
- Bisphenol-A is found to be **estrogenic.**

Remedies for not bonding

- Use acid-etching techniques
- Use sandwich technique (combination of GIC and composite resins)
- Use compomers

Acid etching: Mechanical bonding and retention is achieved by applying 30–50% phosphoric acid for 20 sec, and flushed with distilled water. Dissolution of phosphates causes micro-pores. Thin bonding agents or restoratives applied, flow into these, and set forming micro-tags which cause mechanical bonding (for dentin bonding only 10% acid is used).

54. Varieties of composite restorative resins

- **Chemically cured:** Dispensed as two pastes-now becoming rare
- **UV cured composites:** Replaced by VLC, due to health hazards, low depth of curing, gradual decrease of UV intensity, long warming up time, expensive source, etc.
- **VLC composites:** Dispensed as single paste in different shades: Most common due to command setting, greater depth of curing, less wastage, no health hazards, constant intensity (and setting times), simpler and cheaper source.
- **Anterior, posterior, universal, VLC composites**
- **Hybrid posterior composites: Stronger, due to more fillers of different sizes**
- **Flowable:** Less and smaller fillers and thinner resins—for pit and fissures, etc.
- **Preventive restorative resins:** Microfilled—thin flowable with bonding agents.
- **Glaze composites:** Thin, with less or zero fillers, applied over hybrid or large particle composites.
- **Packable:** Paste like consistency for easy condensation.
- **Prosthodontic composites:** Direct technique: Apply agar separating medium, prepare inlays or onlays on the prepared tooth, polymerise, remove from tooth, finish it and then cement.
- **Prosthodontic composites**—Indirect technique: Inlays or onlays are prepared in clinical laboratory on the die from the impression of prepared tooth, heat cured (at 140°C

and 0.6 bar pressure for 10 min), or light cured, finished and then cemented. (1 bar= 1 atm=14.5 psi=32 inches or 76 cm height of mercury column.

55. Pit and fissure sealants: Preventive resin restorations.

Pits and fissures are the small crevices in the enamel and sometimes extending to dentin, *usually located at the junction of development grooves.*

Requirements

- Should chemically bond with tooth structure.
- Chemically stable, i.e. biocompatible.
- Sufficient mechanical properties.
- High flow and wetting properties, i.e. low surface tension
- Low viscosity and low or zero angle of contact.
- COTE should be similar (i.e. 11.4 ppm/°C) to tooth.
- Good insulators of heat and electricity.
- Match with the tooth colour.

Materials used

- Glass-ionomer cements–type III (which can bond chemically, has low COTE) and anticariogenic
- Composite resins (micro filled-flowable composites)–with less amount of fillers.

Bonding agents: *Refer* to section A, MCQs 10-1 to 10-16

6. Silver Amalgam Alloys

56. Low copper silver amalgam alloy—lathe cut powder particles with triple distilled arsenic free mercury

Amalgamation is done only by **triturating** as Hg does not wet the particles due to oxide layer, high surface tension (465 dynes/cm) and large angle of contacts (135°).

On triturating: (Hg/alloy = 50–54%, for increasing dryness or 1:1 by wt, for Eame's techniques).

$$Ag\text{-}Sn(\beta) + Ag_3Sn\ (\gamma) + Hg \rightarrow$$
$$Ag^2Hg_3(\gamma_1) + Sn_7Hg\ (\gamma_2) + \text{unreacted}\ (\beta, \gamma + Hg)$$

Table 2.6.1: Compositions: Low copper silver amalgam alloys		
Composition	*Wt %*	*Functions*
Silver	65–68	Forms β and γ phases of Ag-Sn which helps amalgamation
Tin	26–29	Decreases corrosion resistance, strength cause dimensional changes and increase creep
Copper	3–6	(< 13%)—helps comminution or cutting.
Zn	1–2%	Scavenger, increase brittleness, delayed expansion, corrosion.

Properties

Compressive strength (1 hour): Low, 145 MPa, after 1 week, = 300 MPa.

Tensile strength: 50–60 MPa, in 24 hours.

Creep: High, 1–2%, causes marginal breakdown.

Modulus of elasticity: 40,000 to 80,000 MPa after 1 week, depending on rate of loading.

Surface hardness: 110 to 120 KHN after 1 week.

COTE: High = 25 ppm/°C, causes percolation and marginal or microleakage.

Uses

- Used as posterior restorative materials in high stress bearing areas.

Disadvantages

- Low 1 Hr strength (145 MPa)
- Zinc containing alloys cause-delayed expansion and corrosion.
- Inability to chemically bond with the tooth structure,
- Metallic lustre-poor aesthetics.
- Mercury health hazards
- High conductivity causes thermal and galvanic shocks (Remedy: Use insulating base)
- Large cavity with undercut required, needs removal of more tooth material

- Large creep and COTE cause marginal breakdown and microleakage

Microstructure: γ_1 and γ_2 crystals grow, binding the unreacted particles $(\beta + \gamma) + Hg$

57. High copper silver amalgam alloy powder, dispensed as dispersed (admix) or single composition lathe-cut and spherical powder particles (Ag-Cu eutectic alloy)

Disperse alloy (sometimes dispensed in proportioned capsules).

Composition: 1 part of spherical-silver + copper (72:28) eutectic alloy, with 2 parts of low copper lathe cut alloys.

Approximately

Silver = 50–60%, Tin = 20–25%, Copper = 13–30% (> 13%), and Zn = 1–2% (Functions are same as in item 56).

Amalgamation: On triturating with mercury (Hg: Alloy = 48–50%)

$$Ag\text{-}Sn(\beta) + Ag_3Sn(\gamma) + Ag_3Cu2(\epsilon) + Hg \rightarrow Ag_3Hg_2(\gamma_1) + (Cu_6Sn_5) + \text{unreacted } (\beta, \gamma, \epsilon + Hg)$$

Micro structure

- The γ_1 and η phases crystallize, separately binding unreacted particles. This did not improve the one hour strength and resistance to creep.

Compressive strength: 130–140 MPa (in 1 hour), and after 1 week = 400 MPa.

Tensile strength: 45–55 MPa (24 hours)

Creep: 0.5–1.0%

Modulus of elasticity: 40,000–80,000 MPa.

Surface hardness: 110–120 KHN.

COTE: 25–50 ppm/°C.

All almost similar to low copper amalgam

58. High copper single composition silver amalgam alloy— dispensed as fine grain lathe cut powder

Composition: Silver = 45–60%, Tin = 15–25%, Copper = 13–20%, Zn = 0%. These are melted together and lathe cut or spherical particles are prepared. These are kept at 100°C for 24 hours (functions of these are same as in Table 2–23).

Amlgamation reaction:

$$Ag\text{-}Sn(\beta) + Ag_3Sn(\gamma) + Cu_3\,Sn + Hg \rightarrow Ag_3Hg_2(\gamma_1) + \eta$$
$$(Cu_6Sn_5) + unreacted\text{-}\beta + \gamma + Cu_3\,Sn + Hg$$

Microstructure: The *prismatic phase crystals grow interconnecting and intermeshing with* γ_1 *crystals* and bind unreacted particles. Due to this, it has

- **Low** Hg/Alloy ratio = 45–50%.
- **High 1 hr compressive strength** = 260–270 MPa, and restoration can be completed in single sitting.
- **Higher maximum** strength = 510 MPa,
- **Higher TS:** 65–70 MPa (24 hours)
- **Lowest creep:** 0.05–0.1%.

59. Copper amalgam (anti bacterial), dispensed as pellets containing Hg (out dated)

Compositions: Cu = 30–40% and Hg = 60–70%.

Manipulation: These pellets are heated in steel spatula (scoop) until the mercury droplets come out to the surface, triturated and condensed into the cavity. Earlier, used for deciduous teeth in rampant caries due to antibacterial effect of copper. But nowadays not used due to low corrosion resistance, poor mechanical properties and large excess of Hg.

60. Gallium alloys

Gallium (density = 5.9 gm/cc and melting at 29.8°C) replaces Hg.

Compositions

Powder has Ag = 50%, Sn = 25%, Cu = 15%, Pd = 9%, etc.

Liquid has Ga = 65% and, In, Sn, etc., which depress melting temperature of Ga. On trituration, the Ga alloys formed bind the unreacted powder particles. Ga is more cytotoxic, cause adverse effects on pulp and mix becomes too thin and difficult to condense.

61. Indium containing amalgam

Indium content in mercury of high copper silver alloy is increased up to 40%. This shows many favorable properties which are under investigations. However more attention is given to develop hybrid VLC composite resins due to their additional aesthetic qualities.

62. Manipulation of silver amalgam alloys with mercury

Steps followed: Selection criteria, proportioning (Hg/alloy), triturating, squeezing, mulling, condensing (homogeneously by 1.6 kg force), carving, finishing (burnishing—polishing).

Instruments used

- Glass mortar and pestle or amalgamator
- Amalgam and plastic mix carriers
- Amalgam condenser (round, rectangular)
- Carvers—diamond, Wartz' and Hollenback
- Ball and T-burnishers
- Matrix band retainers (numbers 1 and 8), and polishing rubber cups

63. Amalgam bond

Material used

- The 4-META (methacryloxyethy trimellitate anhydride) resin was found to have large bond strength with metal alloys and silver amalgam which improves mechanical retention.
- Bonding of fresh amalgam to old amalgam restoration in the repairing procedures is not successful.

7. Auxiliary Materials, Waxes, Investments in Casting

64. Modelling wax or base plate waxes, dispensed as rectangular sheets of 15 cm length, 10 cm width, and 0.15 cms thickness.

Causes for distortion: Relaxation of internal stresses induced during manipulation due to high COTE and low thermal conductivity.

Table 2.7.1: Compositions of modelling waxes		
Ingredients	*Wt%*	*Functions*
Ceresin wax	80	Improves carving characteristics
Bees wax	12	Reduces brittleness and flow at mouth temperature and gives glossiness.
Natural or synthetic resin	3	Gives stable flow properties
Microcrystalline wax	2–5	Establishes required melting points

Precautions (remedies) to minimize wax distortions

- Air should not be incorporated
- Homogenous softening is required
- Increments should be properly bonded
- Artificial teeth should be carefully sealed
- Do not delay curing for long time.

Uses

- To make occlusal rims for establishing the vertical dimensions, the plane of occlusion and initial arch forms in complete denture fabrications.
- To produce the desired contour of the denture after teeth is set in position.
- To make patterns for orthodontic appliances and prosthesis, other than complete dentures.
- To check various articulating relations in the mouth and to transfer them to mechanical articulators.

65. Beading and boxing waxes, provided as rods and sheets of about 10 cm lengths

Manipulation

- The impression is contoured with *beading wax rod* of thickness about 3 mm and then *boxing wax sheet* of about 3 cm width.
- The stone mix is poured to cover the teeth portion and vibrated.
- Remaining mix or fresh plaster mix is poured and allowed to set.

Uses: For beading and boxing for obtaining desired contours of the gypsum products casts and bases.

66. Sticky wax—*model cement*—supplied as small yellow colored rods or sticks.

- **Compositions—**Bees' wax, synthetic and natural resins like gum dammer, etc.
- At room temperature it is hard, and brittle when heated, it becomes tacky or sticky.
- This is sometimes called model cement.

Uses

- To join the parts of crown and bridge initially on the cast before soldering.
- In denture repair procedures, it is melted and poured into the gap between the parts of broken denture mounted on the cast. During acrylisation, this is removed by flushing with hot water, and then replacing by acrylic dough.

67. Carving wax: Supplied as rectangular blocks

Uses: For practising carving anatomical features of teeth and preparing model patterns.

67a. Casting wax: Supplied as very smooth thin square pieces or preformed into various designs (laces, saddles. clasps of different sizes)

Use: For preparing smooth wax patterns for RPDS of hard PBM alloys to minimize trimming and finishing.

68. Inlay waxes: Supplied as deep blue or purple blocks, rods or sticks of about 7.5 cm long and 3 mm in diameter.

Classifications

- **Type I:** Medium wax (for direct technique—inside the mouth)
- **Type II:** Soft waxes (for indirect technique—outside the mouth on the die)

Causes for distortion: Internal stress relaxations due to:

- Nonuniform heating while softening.
- Improper bonding of increments.

Table 2.7.2: Compositions		
Ingredients	*Wt%*	*Functions*
Paraffin wax	60	It is used to establish melting point
Carnauba wax	20	Increases melting range, decreases flow at mouth temperature
Ceresin wax	5	Improves carving characteristics of the wax
Gum dammar	3	Improves smoothness, and resistance to chipping
Bees wax	5	Reduces flow at mouth temperature and reduces brittleness
Synthetic resins	2	Gives suitable flow properties to the wax

- Applying non-uniform pressure during cooling
- Addition of molten waxes to areas of deficiency, introduces stresses during cooling
- During manipulation and cooling, wax molecules get displaced and the stresses induced, relax causing distortion.
- Removal of wax pattern carelessly (apply a drop of lubricant earlier),
- Delay in investing, (if unavoidable, store in cold water or refrigerator for short time) **(Remedies are suggestive)**

Uses: For preparing wax patterns for inlays; onlays, crown and bridges, and sprue former in lost wax casting procedure.

69. Sprue former

Spruc is thc channel or ingate to thc mould of thc wax pattern invested in the casting ring, to allow the molten wax to drain out and molten alloy liquid to enter and completely fill the mould space. Thin vent sprues used to drive away air trapped in mould.

Materials used

- Special wax supplied as rope form (rolls) of different diameters (gauges) for selection.

- Hollow stainless steel wires of different diameters and lengths. These are to be coated with thin layer of *inlay wax* by dipping in molten wax.

70. Cross-section diagram of invested and divested casting ring/cross-section of invested casting ring after wax burn-out. (*Note: This model is prepared for study purpose ref diagram*)

8. Investment Materials

These are *refractory mould materials* used in casting procedures (for classification and requirements, *refer* to MCQs 15-1 to 15-22).

71. Gypsum bonded investment material (GBIM): Rarely used nowadays

Table 2.8.1: Compositions		
Powder	%	*Functions*
Refractory materials – Quartz, crystobalite, tridymite or mixture	60–80	Increases strength porosity, thermal stability, and expansion
Binder—type III dental stone	15–30	Increases strength, porosity and expansion
Modifiers—Na, K, Li chlorides	1–10	Prevents shrinkage
Reducing agents— Cu, graphite colour	2–3	Prevent oxidation of alloy surfaces

Setting action

When, weighed amount of powder and measured volume of water are mixed, the calcium sulphate dihydrates formed sets and binds the refractory particles forming a *porous* mould mass.

Setting reaction:

$2CaSO_4.\frac{1}{2} H_2O + 3H_2O \rightarrow 2CaSO_4.2H_2O + Heat$

Setting time: 5–25 min (ADA)

Compressive strength: = >2.4 MPa. in 2 hrs.

Equation for compensation of casting shrinkage:

Wax shrinkage + Alloy shrinkage = Total shrinkage = Setting expansions (by NSE or HSE) + Thermal expansions. (High heat = 600°C or low heat = 400°C, methods)

Advantages

- Adequate strength, porosity, controllable setting and thermal expansions and simple methods of manipulation.

Disadvantages

- Cannot withstand high casting temperatures, due to disintegration

  Above 600°C, $CaSO_4 + C \rightarrow CaO + SO_2\uparrow + CO\uparrow$
  Above 1000°C, $CaSO_4 \rightarrow CaO + SO_2\uparrow + O_2\uparrow$
- SO_2 causes discoloration of HN, N alloys
- Hygroscopic material—has short shelf life.
- Too high casting force and rapid heating can fracture investment (cause fins)
- Cannot be used for high fusing alloys of Pd, base metals and titanium. Hence phosphate bonded investment is used nowadays

72. Phosphate bonded investment material (PBIM)-dispensed as powder in sachets and freeze-free colloidal silica liquids

Table 2.8.2: Compositions		
Powder	%	*Functions*
Refractory material: Quartz, tridymite crystobalite or their mixtures	80%	Withstand high temperatures, gives large setting (NSE, HSE) expansions
Binder: Mixture of basic MgO and acidic $NH_4H_2PO_4$	20%	Increases strength, setting and thermal expansions
Small amounts of carbon	–	Sometimes, acts as reducing agent
Colloidal silica liquid:	Liquid suspension or freeze stable products, in water to increase setting and thermal expansions	

Setting reactions: *When the powder is mixed with water, it forms.*

$NH_4H_2PO_4$ + MgO + $5H_2O$ → $MgNH_4PO_4.6H_2O$ or $[MgNH_4PO_4.6H_2O]n$ in colloidal multimolecular form, which binds the refractory materials with NSE and HSE.

Thermal changes

On heating above 160°C, it gives $NH_4MgPO_4.H_2O$ + $5H_2O$. Between 300 and 650°C, it gives $(Mg_3P_2O_7)$ + $NH_3\uparrow$
Above 1040°C, it becomes $Mg_3(P_2O_5)_2$

Advantages

- Adequate strength, *>4.8MPa* in 2 hours (ADA specification)
- Large normal hygroscopic setting and thermal expansions (controlled by colloidal silica liquid), to compensate larger casting shrinkages (2.3–2.7%) in base metal alloys casting procedure.
- Thermally stable up to 1040°C.

Disadvantages

- Inadequate porosity *(Use vent sprues)*
- Strong adhesion to PBM alloy castings (require sand blasting),
- Cannot be used for titanium alloy castings.

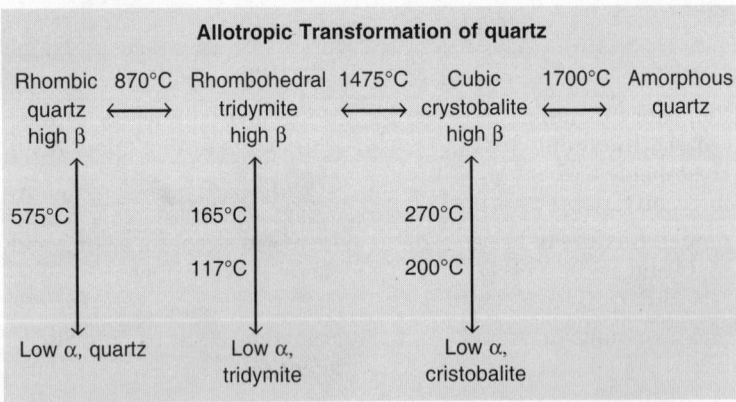

Thermal expansions when heated to about 600°C, Quartz = 1.4%, Tridymite = 1.0%, Cristobalite = 1.8%, Amorphous quartz = negligible.

73. Ethyl silicate-bonded investment material: Supplied as powder of quartz or crystobalite and two liquids or one liquid amine system.

Setting action

- The ethyl silicate is first hydrolyzed into silicic acid which is made to undergo gelation in presence of HCl (and MgO) or certain amines. When the gel investment is heated to about 170°C, alcohol and water vapours escape causing *large green shrinkage* and hard solid mass of *crystobalite refractory non-porous nonconducting material* is formed.

$$Si(OC_2H_5)_4 + 4H_2O \rightarrow Si(OH)_4 + 4C_2H_5OH\uparrow$$

$$nSi(OH)_4 \xrightarrow{\text{heat } 168°C} [-Si-O-Si-O-Si-] \text{ cristobalite} + nH_2O\uparrow$$

Advantages

- The final set mass is entirely crystobalite (a three dimensional -Si-O-Si-O- network) which can withstand very high temperatures even beyond 1150°C. Hence this can be used for high fusing PBM alloys.
- Large thermal expansion compensates *green shrinkage* and also large casting shrinkages.

Disadvantages

- *Nonporous* material requires suitable vent—sprues.
- Complicated investing procedure with vibration, tamping, etc. setting to very hard material
- *Inflammable alcohol vapours* in the laboratory.
- Cannot be used for titanium and its alloys as silica (SiO_2) can oxidize titanium or its alloys easily.

74. Other investment materials

- Soldering investment—should not expand—GBIM
- Divesting investment—large expansions—PBIM
- Ceramming investment—should not expand—GBIM or PBIM
- Ti-alloy casting investments—PBIM-containing Al_2O_3, ZrO_2, MgO, refractory materials and not SiO_2 (which easily oxidises Ti alloys)

9. Metallurgy: Casting Alloys and Techniques

75. Terminologies used

- **Metals > 85 in number: Solidify by super cooling** have free electrons-bonding-ductility, malleability, high conductivity, reflect light—metallic lustre, single melting temperatures, become +ve ion, etc.
- **Alloys or solid solutions:**formed as per Hume-Rothery conditions (*refer* to MCQ 16-8).

Types

- Substitution, disordered, ordered, intermetallic, interstitial, eutectic, etc. have higher strength, lower ductility, and ranges of melting temperature.
- **Alloy phase refers to** physically distinct, mechanically separable, homogeneous portion of solid solution.
- **Constitutional-equilibrium phase diagrams** of solidus-liquidus refers to the entire range or system of the alloys.

76. Classifications of dental casting alloys according to, nobility

- High noble alloys containing gold >40% and noble metals. >60% (major element, Au).
- Noble alloys containing noble metals >25% (major element, Pd or Ag).
- Predominantly base metal PBM alloys contain noble metals, 0–25% (Cr, Co, Ni, Be, Mn, C etc. or Ti, Ni, Al, V etc).
- Noble metals are-Au, Pt, Pd, Rh, Ru, Ir, Os, (Ag is not considered since it undergoes tarnish and corrosion in oral cavity).

Fusion temperature of HN, N, and PBM alloys

- High moble alloys = 870–960°C.
- Noble alloys = 870–1020°C.
- PBM alloys: Type 1 = 1275–1300°C, Type 2 = >1300°C

77. High noble (HN) casting alloys supplied as pellets

Approximate properties of HN and metal alloys: *Refer to* Table 2.9.1.

Uses: Metal ceramics, all metal castings, resin veneering and RPD frameworks.

Table 2.9.1: Compositions and alloying properties of HN alloys

Contents	%	Functions—alloying properties.
Gold >40% (noble metals >60%)	40–80	Increases corrosion resistance and highly biocompatible
Silver (has corrosion resistance with Pd)	10–25	Alloying with copper—lowers melting point and increases hardness (solution hardening and eutectic alloy formation)
Copper	6–15	Increases strength by precipitation, solution hardening and eutectic alloy formation with silver and decreases melting temperatures to facilitate casting and soldering, C. resistance
Palladium, platinum	1–4	Increase strength, density MP, and decreases COTE as required for metal ceramic bonding and platinum makes the gold alloys white
Zinc	Small amounts	Scavenger, sweeps out oxygen absorbed by molten alloy liquid and reduces gas inclusion porosity in casting
Indium, gallium, iridium	Trace metals	Indium replaces zinc for scavenger. Oxides of gallium formed helps to chemically bond the cast alloys with ceramic Iridium causes greater nucleation and grain refinement of gold alloys.

78. PBM casting alloy pellets—stellites (silver color)—Ni-Cr/ Co-Cr/Ti alloys. (Many trade names—Vitallium, Nobilium, ticonium, etc.)

Uses: Fabrication of indirect restorations such as inlays, onlays, all metal crowns and bridges removable partial denture frame works, metal copings for metal ceramic restoration, etc.

Table 2.9.2: General compositions of PBM alloys Ni-Cr-Mo, Ni-Cr-Mo-Be, Co-Cr-Mo, and Co-Cr-W, etc.		
Contents	%	*Functions*
Co = 0–65%, Ni = 0–80%, or Co + Ni = 65–80%	60–70	Suitable mechanical + thermal properties
Chromium	12–30	Passivating film, solution hardener
Mo-W	5–10	Hardeners and grain refiners
Al, Fe, Cu, Be	0.1–1.5	SolLution hardener and grain refiner
Mn, Si, B	0.1–3	Scavengers, cause brittleness
Sn	Trace	Metal ceramic bonding through tin oxide
Carbon	0.2–0.5	Effective hardener by carbide precipitations in inter-dendritic and inter-granular spaces

79. Low fusing noble metal casting alloys

Compositions: Silver = 40–70%, Palladium = 5–60%, Gold = 0–40%, Copper = 8–14%, and trace elements: Ga, In, Zn (scavengers), Ir (grain refiner), etc.

Aproximate melting temperature ranges: 870–950°C. Alloying and other properties are similar to HN alloys (*refer to* Table 2.9.3.

80. Alpha Titanium (α-Ti)-casting alloy pellets

Titanium undergoes passivation in nano-seconds, by forming impervious protective film of Ti)$_3$ (also *refer* to 87).

This popular light metal has two allotropic forms,

α titanium (HCP) → 885°C → β titanium (BCC)

Compositions: CpTi has Fe, O, N, C, as trace impurities (accordingly, grades 1,2,3,4,5,7 and their UTS varies from 240 to 600 MPa. Casting α titanium alloys contain, Al, Sn, Zr (as α-stabilisers).

Approximate properties

Density: 4.51 gm/cc (*very low, centrifugal casting force is not sufficient*)

Table 2.9.3: Properties (approximate value-ranges)

Properties	FEM casting alloys			PBM orthodontic—wires			Noble metal
	Cr-Co alloys	Cr-Ni alloys	Cr-Co-Ni, alloys	18–8 stainless steel	β Titanium	Nickel-Titanium	Pd-Ag, etc. alloys
Yield strength, YS (MPa)	470–535	250–500	300–510	1600	930	430	250–450 Quenched
UTS (MPa)	600–850	500–800	550–820	2100	1275	1400	700–1150
Mod. of elasticity (MPa)	225,000	180,000	210,000	200,000	71,700	41,400	90,000–110,000
Surface hardness (KHN)-quenched	350–415	230–335	300–370	250–350	210	270	140–230
Fusion temperature—middle of ranges	1300–1500°C	1275–1300°C	1300–1450C	1240–1260°C	1660°C	1350—1450°C	900–1100°C

Casting α Titanium has YS = 430MPa TS = 700 MPa, MOE = 117,000 MPa.

Ortho wire β Titanium has yield strength = 930 MPa TS = 1275 MPa, MOE = 71,700 MPa.

Melting temperature (CpTi) = 1668°C, COTE = 9.4 ppm/°C.

Disadvantages: Problems in casting Ti alloys

- High fusion temperature, very low density (4.51 gm/cc) and high oxygen sensitivity. Hence the alloy is melted in vacuum by electric arc, and casting is done under argon gas pressure, centrifugal machine (with suction and compressions).
- Special phosphate bonded investment material with refractory materials, Al_2O_3, ZrO_2, MgO, ZrO and their combinations are used.

Uses

- Casting of crowns, bridges, RPD frameworks, material of choice for implants, etc. due to its bioactivity.
- Preparation of metallic restorations from metal blocks by CAD-CAM and copy-milling techniques.

81. Technique alloy pellets—Japanese gold, Bronze, Goldent-nonprecious gold

- **Composition:** Cu = 54%, Zn = 34% and Al = 12%
- **Aproximately—melting temperature ranges** 750–850°C
- **Density:** 8.0–8.2 gm/cc
- **Disadvantages**: Low corrosion resistance and strength.
- **Uses:** Used as an economical substitute for gold alloys in preclinical teaching situations and now outdated due to very low corrosion resistance.

82. Casting crucibles

For low fusing (HN and N alloys), high fusing HN, N, and PBM alloys, of clay, silica, zircon, graphite inserts.

83. Alternatives to metal casting techniques

- CAD-CAM procedure (chair side technology)
- Copy milling
- Electroforming,
- Sintering of burnished foil techniques, etc.

84. Casting defects and remedies: Refer to MCQs

Types of casting defects

- Distortion, i.e. change in shape or in size or both cause misfit
- Discoloration by $SO_2\uparrow$ of gypsum bonded investments
- Surface roughness, unevenness, and nodules
- Internal porosities—solidification shrinkage and gas inclusion
- Incomplete castings, back pressure porosities.
- Fins

10. Wrought Alloys used in Orthodontia

85. Carbon steels and stainless steels

Ferritic (bcc), austenitic (fcc), cementite, pearlite, martensitic, (distorted monoclinic or HCP), etc., refer to MCQs 20-1 to 20-15.

- Ferritic stainless steel contains, Cr = 11.5–27%, Ni-0%, C = 0–2%, Mn = 2%. This has adequate corrosion resistance at low temperature, used for machine parts, large equipment, sheets, in industries.
- Martensitic stainless steel contains Cr = 11.5–17%, Ni = 0–2.5%, C = 0.15–1.2%., Fe =balance. Formed by diffusionless transformation from austenite when quenched. This has high surface hardness = 1200 KHN. Blades of cutting steel instruments are hardened by controlled quenching (martensite formation).

86. *18-8 austenitic stainless steel* **orthodontic wire for passive appliances**

Approximate properties (almost same)
- **Melting temperature ranges:** 1240°–1260°C
- **MOE:** 200,000 MPa
- **Surface hardness:** 250–400 KHN
- **Density:** 8.5 gm/cc
- **Yield strength:** 1100–1750 MPa
- **Ultimate tensile strength: 2,200** MPa

Table 2.10.1: Compositions of austenitic and 18–8 stainless steels

	Austenitic %	18–8%	Functions
Chromium	16–26	18	Imparts strength, hardness and corrosion resistance by passivation
Nickel	7–22	8	Prevents the formation martensite phase during cooling depresses martensite formation temperature
Mn or Mo	2–5	2	Increases strength and retains ductility and malleability
Carbon	< 0.25	0.15	Very effective hardener
Iron	Balance (70–80)	Balance (70%)	Impart strength, ductility, malleability, etc.

Corrosion of stainless steels

Passivation: Attaining good corrosion resistance by formation of a thin film of chromic oxide on the surface which is impervious to oxygen.

Sensitization: Loss of corrosion resistance, when heated above 400°C. Then the carbon atoms diffuse and reduce chromium oxide to $(CrFe)_4C$, causing loss of corrosion resistance.

Stabilization of 18-8 stainless steel: By adding *niobium, titanium and tantalum* about six times carbon, diffusions of carbon atoms are temporarily arrested and corrosion resistance is not lost during quick heating.

Weld-decay: Loss of corrosion resistance by prolonged overheating while welding.

Uses: For orthodontic passive (reactive) and active appliances, bands.

87. β Titanium-orthodontic wires (also *refer* to Question 80)

Allotropic forms: α titanium (HCP) ← 885°C → β titanium (BCC).

Compositions: CpTi has Fe, O, N, C, as trace impurities (grades 1,2,3,4,5,7) with UTS = 240–600 MPa. β Titanium alloys contain, Mo, V, Ta (β-stabilisers), common alloy(TMA) has Ti = 79%, Mo = 11%, Zr = 6%, Sn = 6%.

Approximate properties

- Density-4.51 gm/cc *(very low, hence centrifugal casting force is not sufficient)*
- α titanium has yield strength (YS) = 430 MPa TS = 700 MPa, MOE = 117,000 MPa), used for casting implants
- β Titanium has yield strength (YS) = 430 MPa, TS = 700 MPa, MOE = 117,000 MPa, used as orthodontic wire for activation.
- Melting temperature (CpTi) = 1668°C.
- COTE = 9.4 ppm/°C
- Bio compatible

88. Ni-Ti: Super elastic nitinol (Ni-Ti), orthodontic wires, dispensed as arch-wires of transformation temperatures 25°C, 35°C, 45°C, etc.

Graph: Super elasticity of nitinol wire (*refer* to Color Plate 41 and Fig. 72).

Composition: This is an equi-atomic (1:1 atomic ratio) alloy of nickel (54%) and titanium (44%), with 2% of Co, Cr, or Cu. This has two allotropic forms—austenitic (HCP) below 885°C and martensite (BCC) above. These can also be induced by stresses.

Properties

- Good biocompatibility
- The transformation takes by *twinning which is diffusionless deformation* to form mirror-like images of atoms in lattice.
- *Super-elasticity*: Additional expansions on heating or reducing shear stress or contraction during cooling and increasing stress due to allotropic changes (at TTR)
- *Shape memory:* Recovering earlier shape due to reversal of twinning below TTR.

MOE: 41,400 MPa (lowest of all alloys and highest flexibility).

YS: 930 MPa (high) which gives *large elastic range or flexibility.*

TS: 1,400 MPa (large resilience).

Uses: Active orthodontic wire appliances, endodontic flexible files.

Advantages: It has all the properties desired for *active orthodontic appliances,* applying small constant forces for long time.

Disadvantages
- Cannot be soldered or welded but can be joined by using mechanical crimps.
- Patient cannot bear the large pain during quick reversal of twinning.

89. Aesthetic orthodontic wire

Optiflex aesthetic ortho wire.
- **Teflon resin coated NiTi, or β Ti wires:** These have suitable mechanical properties for activation, chemical stability and better aesthetics.
- **Optiflex—glass-fibre reinforced thermoplastic wires:** This has fine glass-fibre ceramic core wire with a translucent *aramid resin,* which is then covered by *candidate resin* like *polycarbonates, polyethylene tetra phthalate glycol.* It is also protected by *transparent nylon,* which acts as *strain retainer.* This can be softened by warming above the Tg of resin.

Disadvantages: Both prevent the movement of teeth, by the friction between wire and bracket.

11. Soldering, Brazing and Welding

90. *Soldering* is a metal joining technique using low fusing fillers of liquidus temperatures <450°C. Soft solders—Plumber's solder—has eutectic—lead–tin alloy = 2:3 ratio. Fusion temp = about 260°C. Has low strength, and poor corrosion resistance.

Brazing refers to hard gold and silver solders, whose liquidus temperatures are above 450°C.

Table 2.11.1: Compositions		
Ingredients	*Gold solders, wt. %*	*Silver solders, wt. %*
Gold	45–85	–
Silver	8–30	10–80
Copper	8–20	15–50
Zinc	2–4	5–35
Tin	2–4	–
Cadmium	3–5	Small amount
Phosphorous	–	Small amount

Properties

Gold solders: UTS = 220–300MPa (heat treated = 430–630 MPa), Fusion temperature ranges = 700—820°C, good resistance to corrosion.

Silver solders: UTS = 240–320 MPa, fusion temperatures = 600–700°C, slightly lower corrosion resistance.

91. Soldering fluxes and antifluxes

Fluxes: Used to wet the surface of the basis (or parent) metals, and increase the flow of molten solders.

These are supplied as powder/paste forms or included in hollow solder wires.

- Type-1: Protective fluxes (borax),
- Type-2: Reducing fluxes ($Na_2B_2O_7.10\ H_2O$ or borax flux),
- Type-3: Dissolving fluxes (fluorides) used while soldering base metal alloys.

Compositions

Borax fluxes: Borax = 55, boric acid = 35 and silica = 10 parts, are used for HN and N alloys.

Fluoride fluxes: KF or NaF = 50–60%, boric acid = 25–30%, K_2CO_3 or Na_2CO_3 = 8–10%, are used for base metal alloys.

Antifluxes: Marking with lead pencil or applying rouge or whitting ($CaCO_3$) to prevent the flow of molten solder to undesired areas.

Melting heat sources: Natural, butane, propane, hydrogen, or oxyacetylene, gas (reducing pale blue) flames, electrical resistance heaters or lasers.

Precautions: Minimum gap distance, minimum time taken to melt solder and soldering procedures.

Techniques: Free hand soldering, investment soldering

92. Soldering investment materials supplied in powder form.

Requirements: Should not undergo setting or thermal expansions, which may distort the appliances and thermal stability.

Use: To avoid the distortion of long span bridges and RPD frameworks during fabrication, which are cast in separate parts and then joined by brazing, welding, or metal joining techniques, by investing technique.

Outline of procedure: The parts to be joined should be assembled on master casts, joined with molten sticky wax, and then invested on a tile. After eliminating the sticky wax, suitable fluxes and anti-fluxes are used. Molten solder is poured into the gap (Fig. 74).

93. *Welding*: Refers to metal joining by locally fusing and pressing with or without a third brazer alloy.

Methods: Gas welding, arc welding, spark welding, electrical welding, infrared ray welding, and laser welding (*refer* to 86).

Precautions: Quick melting and welding to avoid formation of other weaker intermetallic alloys, and weld decay (failure of welded joints of 18–8 stainless steels due to sensitisation—loss of corrosion resistance when heated above 400°C).

Other methods of metal joining: Cast joining, casting to embedded alloys.

12. Dental Ceramics and Metal Ceramics

94. Ceramic powder of different shades and opacifiers—dentine (body)/enamel/gingival (cervical)/opaque/glaze varieties, etc.

Ingredients are fritted powdered and dispensed in different shades, opacities and fusion temperatures.

Classifications (refer to MCQ): According to fusion temperature, composition, processing methods, applications, etc.

Table 2.12.1: Compositions

Ingredients	Wt%	Functions
Feldspar soda-$Na_2O.Al_2O_3.6SiO_2$, potash-$K_2O.Al_2O_3.SiO_2$, lime-$CaAl_2O_3.6SiO_2$	60–80	Basic glass former
Alumina-Al_2O_3	8–10	Strengthener, glass former, opacifiers
Kaolin ($Al_2O_3.SiO_2.2H_2O$)	3–5	Binder
Quartz	15–20	Filler
Boric oxide	2–7	Glass former, flux
Oxides of Na, K, Ca	9–15	Glass modifier, interrupter, fluxes
Metallic pigments (oxides of Zn, Sn, Ti)	< 1%	To get different colour shades

Properties of feldspathic porcelains (approximated): Refer to porcelain teeth, Item 27 MCQ

Methods of condensations of ceramic slurry on the platinum foil adapted ceramic die *refer* **to model answers RGHS)**

- Spatulation
- Brush technique
- Vibration method
- Ultrasonic vibrations—transmitted electrically.

In each method, water coming out is removed using blotting paper or linen cloth. This is to minimize firing shrinkage.

Stages of sintering/firing: Temperature of muffle chamber is initially kept at 650°C for 30 mins article is moved inside, and temperature is raised to 950°C in 5 minutes at the rate of 5°C/sec.

- **Low bisque stage:** The surface particles begin to soften and join. There is no volume shrinkage and no cohesion.
- **Medium bisque stage:** On further heating more softening of particles takes place and begin to melt. There is better cohesion and slight volume shrinkage.
- **High bisque stage:** Further heating causes *complete melting* of all particles producing complete cohesion and *maximum volume contraction*.

Pyroplastic flow—on prolonged heating the article looses sharp corners and shape (flow of highly viscous liquid).

Glazing causes smooth, glossy surface and increases flexure strength.

Methods

- **Autoglazing or self glazing**
- **Add on or extended glazing**

Staining: Colour frits of metal oxides are applied to imitate *calcified check-lines* (in natural teeth) before glazing

Methods to compensate, volume shrinkage of 30–40% during firing

- Applying the slurry (more transparent) layer on the fired article and firing again. But repeated firing may reduce the strength.
- Prepares about 13% linear oversized (i.e. 1/3 of 40%) patterns before first firing.
- Firing layer after layer (which also together by mismatching COTE).

Methods to reduce porosity

- Firing under vacuum
- Firing under diffusible gases (H_2 or He)
- Cooling under pressure

The entire procedure is complicated and technique sensitive which demands high skill or training for technicians. Recently simpler sophisticated CAD-CAM procedure is used

95. Toughening of ceramics

Ceramics have oxygen bonding and no free electrons. Hence they are very poor conductors of heat and solidify as vitreous structures with millions of microcracks. These propagate on stressing and cause fractures.

These are toughened by

1. Interruption of crack propagations

- Dispersion toughening—by adding very hard, alumina, crystalline leucite ($K_2O,Al_2O_3.4SiO_2$), lithia di silicate ($LiO_2.2SiO_2$), magnesia, alumina spinnel, zirconia, etc.
- Transformation toughening by including partially stabilized, zirconia.

2. Introduction of residual surface compressive stresses
- *Ion exchange or chemical tempering by replacing* Na ions by larger K ions (immersing in molten KNO_3 solution).
- Thermal tempering (rapid cooling of surface)
- Missmatching of thermal expansions of different layers.

3. *Designing articles without stress raisers,* **i.e.** **avoiding sharp corners and wrinkles.**

96. Crowns, crowns and bridges, metal-ceramic appliances, full metal crowns and bridges (i.e. without ceramic veneer or facing) etc. appliances.

Ideal requirements of metals and ceramics for metal-ceramics: *Refer* to MCQ 17-27.

Bonding mechanisms [high ST (380 dynes/cm at 1100°C), and angle of contact (140°), prevent wetting and bonding].

- *Mechanical:* Metal surface is made rough by using diamond or carbide burs or sand blasting
- *Thermal mismatching* the COTE by 0.5 ppm/°C, which is done by adding Pd, Pt, etc. to reduce COTE of metals to 13.5–14 ppm/°C and raising COTE of ceramics to 13–13.5 ppm/°C by including leucite porcelain or divitrifiers.
- *Chemical bonding:* Through oxygen of the *tin oxide layer* formed on the metal surface.

Metal ceramic bond failures (*refer* to Question 5 on page 233)

- Metal and metal oxide inter-phase—due to poor bonding.
- Within the metal oxide layer—due to thicker weaker oxide layer.
- Metal oxide—ceramic junction—due to weak bonding
- Metal or ceramic regions—due to lower strength than the bond strength.

Advantages of metal ceramics

- High strength and fracture resistance, etc., imparted by the metals.
- Excellent aesthetics imparted by the ceramics.

Disadvantages

- Very complicated fabrication technique.
- Reflection of light from white metal cause *non-vital appearance.* *An opaque ceramic* is first applied and fired, then cervical, dentin, enamel and glaze porcelain, etc. are used.
- Poor aesthetics due to metallic lustre, compared to all-ceramic restorations.
- Removal of more healthy parts of tooth

97. Improvements on metal-ceramic techniques

- Swagged metal foil
- Bonded platinum foil
- Electrodeposition of gold and tin

98. All ceramic restorations

- Castable glasses—DICOR-ceramming—chameleon effect.
- Injection moulding techniques.
- Hot pressing technique.
- CAD–CAM. techniques.

99. Glass infiltrated core ceramics

Core ceramics powder is made into thick slurry applied to a die, slip-casted and partially sintered up to the low bisque stage. Low fusing glass ceramic (sodium-lanthanum glass) mix is applied and fired, when the molten glass enters into the pores thereby reducing the firing shrinkage. This gives higher flexure strengths.

- **Inceram spinnel (ICS)** has MgO, Al_2O_3, core: Translucent-high flexure strength = 400 MPa, used for anterior crowns veneers, inlays, onlays.
- **Inceram alumina (ICA)** has Al_2O_3, core: More opaque, higher flexure strength = 500 MPa, used for posterior crowns, anterior 3-unit FPDs, inlays, onlays.
- **Inceram zirconia (ICZ)** has $Al_2O_3 = 70\%$ and $ZrO_2 = 30\%$, **core.** More opaque, highest flexure strength = 700 MPa, used for posterior crowns, bridges, etc.

100. Artificial porcelain teeth

Fabrication: Pack the high fusing opaque, translucent, more transparent ceramic slurries and color frits, in the 2 or 3 parts of split metal die, dried, fired, finished and glazed.

For properties and comparison (*refer* to MCQ 13-57 and Table 1.13.1)

13. Dental Implant Materials

101. Definitions, indications and contraindications: Refer to MCQs 24.1 to 24-14

Basic components

- **Fixtures:** Grooved, threaded, or perforated implant structures plasma coated with HAP or TCP.
- **Abutments:** Strong connections to fixtures and prosthesis by screwing, cementations, swaging or through internal or external hexagonal structures with antirotation system.
- **Prosthesis-over dentures**

Varieties

- *Epithelial*: Implants are inserted into the oral mucosa
- *Subperiosteal*: Implant metal frames and super structures are placed over jaw-bones
- *Endosteal (endosseous):* Implants are partially submerged in the alveolar or basal bones.
- *Transosteal implants*: Transmandibular implants passing through the entire thickness of alveolar bones.

Materials

Metallic

- Ti alloys, low carbon 18–8 stainless steel, Cr-Co alloys, gold alloys.
- Surface modified or coated with hydroxyapatite (HAP), tri-calcium phosphate (TCP) which improves *osseointegration and bioactivity*

Non-metallic

- Polymer resins, composite, resins
- Inert ceramics: Alumina, zirconia, graphite (do not release ions—gold-standard)
- Bioactive ceramics: HAP, TCP, bioglasses, etc.

102. Hydroxyapatite (HAP) bone graft material in granular or block forms

Uses: *Ridge augmentation or bone graft material,* which acts as skeleton for the formation of new bone structures *by releasing Ca^{++} and PO_4^{---} ions* to the surrounding tissues, which cause *bio-integrations* to the bone, i.e. calcium and phosphorous crystallize locking the collagen fibrils.

14. Mechanics of Cutting, Abrasion and Polishing Tools

103. Hand cutting instruments

Hand cutting instruments have **one or two regular shaped sharp cutting edges** at one end or both ends of the instruments with identification numbers.

Uses: During cavity preparations for restorations to remove unwanted parts by cutting.

Mechanics of cutting, abrasion and finishing

Cutting: The removal of unwanted material with sharp edged, regular shaped, bladed instruments by first applying large compressive force and then shearing to fracture.

Abrasion: Removal of unwanted material from the surface, by grinding or wearing with friction by moving irregularly shaped sharp multi-edged hard particles in unidirection (or chemical corrosion).

Polishing (finishing): Obtaining smooth-glossy micro crystalline surface (Beilby layer) by pressing and moving very fine (F, FF, FFF, or 0, 0, 00 numbered particles in multidirections), or by glazing ceramics, or electropolishing PBM alloys.

104. Classification of dental burs

According to:
- Material of bur heads: Diamond, carbide, steel
- Bur head designs: Round, fissure, inverted cones, and modifications.
- Sizes of cutting bur heads
- Shapes and sizes of cutting edges

Components of burs: Attachment grip, shank, neck, head.

Uses: To cut, round burs for depth, fissure burs for walls and size, inverted cone burs for levelling of floor of cavities.

105. Cross-section of steel burs

Labelled diagrams: *Refer* **to Fig. 83, Color Plate 45**

Identifications: Zero/negative/positive rake angles, tooth angle, clearance angles, radial line, direction of rotation.

106. Cutting efficiency of dental burs is the rate of removal of unwanted material from the work.

This efficiency, i.e. rate of cutting is higher if

- Number of teeth is more,
- Tooth angle is smaller,
- Rake angle is positive and large,
- Optimum clearance angle and chip space.
- Non eccentric to the rotating shaft.
- Least run out.
- Higher speed up to a limit,
- Greater load applied-up to a limit, related to speed
- Use of coolants-water or air spray, which also removes clogging,
- Proper maintenance with frequent lubrications.

107. Surface hardness: It is the resistance to scratching, abrasion, wearing or indentations, determined by Moh's, Brinnel's, Rockwell's, *microhardness by Vicker's, Knoop's methods or using atomic force microscopes.*

108. Abrasives and abrasive agents

(a) Diamond points/discs

Hardness: Synthetic diamond = 5,000–7,000 KHN, natural diamond>10,000 KHN.

Manufacturing: Diamond particles of different sizes (grits) are bonded to the end of the steel shaft through ceramics or *heat resistant polyamides to reduce plucking.* This is *electroplated with nickel and titanium nitride.* Diamond particles of different sizes (grits) are dispersed (bonded) layer by layer to expose maximum area.

Table 2.14.1: Approximate surface hardness of abrasives and materials

Materials	Surface Hardness values (KHN)
Diamond	7000–10,000
Carbides of Si, WB	2400, 2500, 2600
Alumina, emery	1500–2000
Hardened steel	1000–1300
Quartz, silica, etc.	800–820
Ceramics	450–470
Tooth enamel	**340–360**
PBM alloys	250–500
18–8 steel	250–350
HN, N, alloys	120–400
Silver amalgam	110–120
Cementum	**80**
Dentin	**65**
Composite resins	40–50
Gold	25
Acrylics-PMMA	16–20 KHN

Uses: For cutting tooth enamel, shaping carbide and steel burs, reducing PBM appliances and composite resins, GIC restorations, ceramics, etc., (diamond separating discs).

(b) Tungsten carbide burs

Hardness: 2,500KHN

Manufacturing: Tungsten carbide bur is obtained by heating tungsten and graphite powder, at high pressure and temperature, 1500°C. The abrasive powder is *sintered and hot pressed* on the bur head *(powder metallurgy)*. The bur head is shaped using fine diamond points with desired designs like flame, fissure, round, etc.).

Uses: For cutting and abrasions of PBM alloys, ceramics, silver amalgam, composite resins, etc., restorations.

(c) Silicon carbide and carborundum grinding stone, manufacturing: Silicon carbide is bonded to metal shafts,

rotating wheels, grinding stones, etc. through vitreous bonding. The abrasive particles are mixed with ceramics powder slurry with water and cold pressed into metal shanks to form different shapes and sizes. Then it is fired, to fuse the ceramics

Uses: For cutting and trimming and abrading hard PBM alloy, ceramics, appliances, silver amalgam, acrylics, etc.

(d) **Garnet:** Double silicate of Al and one of Fe, Co, Mg, or Mn (hardness = 1300 KHN)—used as coated abrasive and grinding stones

(e) **Zirconium silicates** (hardness = 1200 KHN): Coated abrasive or in prophy pastes

(f) **Quartz and silica varieties** (hardness = around 800 KHN): Common abrasives–bonded to paper, plastic or cloth sheets, marked with grit numbers—40, 60, 80,100, etc. or in powder form.

(g) **Pumice powder:** Siliceous material of *volcanic origin;* hardness = 700–800KHN; fine powder is a common polishing agent.

109. Types of abrasives and tools

- Bonded abrasives: Diamond points, discs, carbide burs; rubber cups, points, etc.
- Coated abrasives: Hard irregular abrasives of different grit sizes (40, 60, 80, 100, 300—with suitable adhesives arc coated on flexible metal discs cellulose, emery (papers), sand (papers), etc.
- Non-bonded abrasives: Fine powders of diamond, carbides, alumina, etc. applied as slurry and alumina particles are used for sand-blasting and air-abrasions
- Grinding and truing stones.

110. Abrasion techniques

- Select suitable abrasives and tools
- Use abrasive particles sizes in descending order
- Move abrasives in one direction
- Apply minimum pressure
- Abraded particle dust should fly away from operator
- Use vacuum suction equipment and mouth-masks

111. Polishing agents supplied in powder form

Polishing refers to smoothening the abraded surface with very fine abrasives (size 0, 00, 000 or F, FF, FFF) or tools, without or with minimum removal of the surface material. The *microcrystalline Beilby layer* formed becomes glossy, reflects or refracts light completely. Polishing agents are supplied in powder form or rubber cups or embedded in wax.

(a) **Synthetic diamond:** Very fine powder of particle size, <10 microns used for polishing very hard metal/alloys.

(b) **Aluminium oxides (hardness = 1000–1500 KHN): For very hard surfaces, sand-blasting, prophy pastes.**

(c) **Tripoli**: Finely powdered porous siliceous rock— polishing agent. For base metals, silver amalgam, composite resin restorations, etc.

(d) **Rouge (pink or red color) powder or in wax block:** For polishing soft metal alloys specially, for gold alloy restorations (and for coloring impression compound).

(e) **French chalk (calcite: $CaCO_3$) whiting** supplied in powder form (SH = 130 KHN) and some time embedded in wax block.

Uses: For polishing direct filling gold (DFG), tooth enamel, amalgam, acrylics and also mild abrasives in dentifrices.

Method of polishing

• The powder is used as slurry in water or glycerin and applied with pressure in multidirections through cotton, silk or felt buffs.

• Apply adequate pressure and move the polishing slurry in multidirections.

• Sometimes, it is bonded to rubber cups and is used for polishing *composite resin, silver amalgams, direct filling gold foil restorations, acrylic resin, etc.*

• *Polishing* points of different sizes and shapes are also available.

• *Microcrystalline Beilby layer* is formed on the substrate in the polishing procedure.

Precautions: While cutting, abrading or polishing of tooth or filling restorations in the oral cavity, temperature rise should be minimized (?)

Other methods of finishing

- Self or add on glazing for ceramics.
- Electropolishing for PBM alloys.
- Apply glaze composites over hybrid or large filler particle composite restorations.

112. Dentifrices supplied in paste form or gel form (powder form now rarely used) in collapsible tubes and also in powder form

Compositions

- Abrasives ($CaCO_3$, CaH_2PO_4, $NaHCO_3$, etc.) = 20–55%
- Detergent—sodium lauryl sulfate = 1–2% (surfactant)
- Humectant (sorbitol, glycerin) = 20–35%
- Demineralized water = 15–25%
- Binder (Carrageenan) = 3%
- Small amounts of tartar controlling agents, fluorides, desensitizers, colors, flavoring agents, etc.

Purpose of using

- Polishing enamel for better esthetics
- Removing food debris, plaque, stained pellicles, micro-organisms and stains to reduce caries, for better hygiene.
- Application of therapeutic materials, like fluorides, desensitizers, tartar controlling agents, etc.

Efficiency of dentifrice depends on abrasivity of dentifrices and the extraoral and intraoral factors. This is measured by finding the radioactive P removed from enamel irradiated by radioactive phosphorus (P).

Prophylactic materials: Hard deposits like plaque, calculus, etc., are the seats for the growth of micro-organisms in the interdental spaces and enhance caries. These are not removed during daily brushing methods. Prophylactic pastes or powders are to be used. These are used in dental clinic and contain harder abrasives like zirconium silicate, alumina, fine silica, etc.

[*Note:* For more viva voce short questions, topics not covered above].

15. Comparison of Human, Acrylic, Porcelain and Composites Resin Teeth

Recent advances in artificial teeth is the development of composite teeth with better mechanical and esthetic properties than auricle teeth. *Refer* to composite resin: *Refer* 47, MCQ 8-96 for comparing properties of restorative cements.

Note: Refer to model questions on long essays, short essays and brief answer types, given at the end of every chapters in *Science of Dental Materials and Clinical Applications*, 3/e (CBS Publisher) by the same author.

Table 2.15.1: Approximate compositions of enamel and dentin

	Mineral phase		Organic phase		Water	
	Vol%	*Wt%*	*Vol%*	*Wt%*	*Vol%*	*Wt%*
Enamel	92	97	2	1	6	2
Dentin	48	69	29	20	23	11

Table 2.15.2: Properties (approximate values) of enamel, dentin, acrylic and porcelain teeth: Also *refer* to MCQ Table 2.15.1

Properties	Enamel	Dentin	Acrylic	Porcelain
Compressive strength (MPa)	380	300	75	170
Tensile strength (MPa)	10	55	65	25, DTS = 35
Modulus of elasticity (MPa)	84,100	18,300	2500	70,000
Surface hardness—KHN (kg/mm^2)	343	68	18–20	460
Shear strength (MPa)	90	135	120	110
Transverse strength (MPa)	–	–	85	140
Modulus of resilience (J/m^3)	0.55	0.94	–	–
Linear COTE. (ppm/°C)	11.4	8.3	80–120	9–12
Thermal conductivity (°C/cm)	0.0022	0.0016	0.006	0.0024

Theory Model Answers for University Examinations

3

The method of presentation of the various aspects of the answers in an organized manner, planning this within the limited time and attempting all the questions, are very important, instead of simply writing the information required. It is better to practice attempting a model question paper before the examination for self assessment, applying all the above principles. In view of this model answers to two university question papers are provided.

According to the duration of examination time, one should distribute the available maximum time according to the marks allotted for each answer. For example, in a three hours question paper comprising two essays carrying 10 marks each, five short essays carrying 5 marks each, 5 brief answers carrying 2 marks each and 15 MCQs of one mark each, the available max time to score one mark is about 180/70, i.e. 2.5 minutes. If only 15 minutes are used for MCQs there is 165/55, i.e. 3 min, to 1 mark. Hence, available max time for an essay is = 30 min (i.e. 5–6 pages), for short essay it is = 15 min (i.e. 2 pages), for brief answer it is 5 or 6 min, (1 page). Complete all the answering little earlier, so that, some time is available for revising and corrections. Watch your watch and strictly adhere to this!

Note: Every answer should have a brief introduction, details as required, applications, conclusions. Numerical values will always enrich your answers. Easily readable clean hand-writing, underlining the keywords, relevant neat diagrams, tabulations, etc. are additional benefits. First read all the questions twice, and plan the extent of answers before proceeding to write. Answer each question within the time limit as mentioned earlier.

YENEPOYA UNIVERSITY
II Year BDS Degree Examinations, November 2015
Time: 3 Hours   Max Marks: 70

DENTAL MATERIALS
QPCODE: 1008

Your answers should be specific to the questions asked.
Draw neat and labeled diagrams wherever necessary.

LONG ESSAYS   **(2 × 10 = 20 Marks)**

1. Classify dental waxes. Describe the composition, properties, manipulation and uses of inlay pattern wax.
2. Classify dental resins and write their ideal requisites. Compare self cure and heat cure acrylic denture base resins. Add a note on repair resins.

SHORT ESSAYS   **(8 × 5 = 40 Marks)**

3. Define dental cast. Write advantages and dis- advantages of gypsum products as cast materials.
4. Condensation silicones *vs* addition silicones.
5. Modifications of GIC.
6. Properties of 18-8 stainless steel.
7. Abrasive agents.
8. Flow and viscosity of dental materials.
9. Fillers and resin matrix in dental composites.
10. Castable ceramics.

SHORT ANSWERS   **(5 × 2 = 10 Marks)**

11. Sprue former.
12. Tray adhesives.
13. Micro-leakage.
14. Gutta-percha.
15. Significance of color in dentistry.

Answers

LONG ESSAYS

1. Classify dental waxes. Describe the composition, properties, manipulation and uses of inlay pattern wax.

Dental waxes are thermoplastic organic polymers, comprising unsaturated hydrocarbons of low molecular weights, about 400 to 4,000 and their derivatives such as some esters, alcohols, free acids, etc. Many varieties of combinations of natural, synthetic, insect and animal origins are used as auxiliary materials in clinics for impressions, bite registrations, and in fabrication procedures of oral appliances.

Classification of dental waxes is required for quick selection of the best materials having desired most suitable properties. Classification is done according to their;

(a) Origin or sources

- *Plants origin:* Carnauba, candelila, cocoa butter, stearic/oleic/palmetic acids, etc. These are microcrystalline waxes.
- *Insects origin:* Beeswax-mixtures of hydrocarbons.
- *Animal origin:* Spermaceti wax.
- *Synthetic waxes:* Very large numbers like esters, polyethylene, glycol, hydrogenated/halogenated waxes, etc.

(b) Applications

- *Pattern waxes:* Modeling-base-plates, casting, preformed waxes, etc.
- *Processing waxes:* Inlay waxes (type 1: medium, type 2: soft): sticky, utility, boxing, beading, carving, etc.
- *Impression waxes:* Corrective impression, bite registration.

Inlay waxes

These are supplied as blue-colored rods of about 7.5 cm length and 3 mm in diameters.

Classifications: Type 1—medium wax for direct patterns and type 2, soft wax for indirect patterns.

Compositions

Ingredients	Wt%	Functions
Paraffin waxes	60	To get thermoplastic properties and softening temperature ranges
Carnauba wax	20	Increases softening ranges, glossiness and decreases flow
Ceresin wax	5	Improves carvability, toughness
Gum dammar	3	Improves smoothness, resistance to flaking and chipping, toughness
Beeswax	5	Controls flow and brittleness
Synthetic resins	2	Stabilize flow properties

Properties

- Low elastic modulus which decreases as temperature rises.
- Flow at 45°C should be between 70% and 90% for both types 1 and 2.
- Hardening temperature ranges for both, are between 40°C and 50°C.
- Large COTE—300–600 ppm/°C cause about 0.3% to 0.4% linear shrinkage of the patterns. Low thermal conductivity cause inhomogeneous solidification and internal stresses which relax and distort the patterns.

Causes for wax distortions and remedies

- Inhomogeneous softening.
- Inadequate bonding between layers.
- Inadequate pressure applied.
- Careless removal of the pattern.
- Relaxation of internal stresses due to delay in investing, (invest the pattern immediately or store in cold water at low temperature for short time).

(**Remedies** are suggestive and write accordingly).

Manipulation

Apply a thin coating of lubricant on the die for easy removal of pattern. Select correct type of wax. Soften the wax rod carefully rotating one end over the blue gas flame. Place molten wax on the die and allow it to harden. Place the next increments before complete hardening, with slight excess. Finally apply adequate pressure while hardening completely. Carve it carefully without flaking, chipping and pulling. Attach the sprue former, remove from the die and invest as early as possible.

Uses: For preparing the accurate wax patterns of inlays, onlays crowns, pontics, bridges, etc., required for the lost wax alloy casting procedures and sometimes for indirect composite resin restorations.

2. Classify dental resins and write their ideal requisites. Compare self cure and heat cure acrylic denture base resins. Add a note on repair resins.

Answer

Classification is required to select the best material—most suitable for the particular clinical conditions.

Classification can be done according to

- *Materials:* Formerly vulcanite, bakelite, cellulose. Now PMMA acrylics (heat, self, or light cure), reinforced acrylics.
- *Moulding techniques:* Compression moulding, injection moulding, fluid-pour and cure resin techniques.
- *Processing (curing) methods:* Heat curing, selfcuring, visible light curing, microwave curing.
- *Applications:* Complete dentures, removable partial dentures, temporary crowns and bridges, denture reliners, denture repairs, maxillofacial reconstructions, orthodontic appliances, athletic mouth protectors.

Ideal requirements of denture base resins

Biological

- Biocompatible, chemically inert, non-allergic, non-carcinogenic, non-irritant, hygienic.

Physical–mechanical

- Low density and light-weight for better retention.
- Dimensional accuracy, and stability for exact fitting.
- Large proportional and elastic limits to resist permanent deformations.

- High compressive, flexure and tensile and impact strengths to resist fractures by dynamic masticating forces.
- High modulus of elasticity to resist deformations.
- Adequate resilience to absorb masticating energies.
- Large abrasive resistance (surface hardness) to resist wearing.
- High fatigue strength and endurance limit for long life.

Thermal
- Low COTE, to resist dimensional contractions during processing
- High thermal conductivity for experiencing real hotness or coldness of foods.
- High softening and distortion temperatures, to resist distortion, in the mouth.

Esthetics
- Transparent or translucent, ability to incorporate suitable color pigments and stability of color parameters.

Others
- Less sophisticated, simple fabricating laboratory techniques without much training or skill, and less expensive.

[*Note:* The most common acrylic denture base materials satisfy only biocompatibility, esthetics and simple techniques but do not satisfy any of the mechanical and thermal requirements.]

Comparison of heat cured and cold cured acrylics

S. No.	Considerations	Heat cured	Cold-self cured
1.	Dispensing/ composition	Powder-liquid	Same
2.	Initiator	Benzoyl peroxide	Same for chemical curing Camphorquinone for VLC
3.	Activator	Heat/micro-waves	Dimethyl paratoluidine/ light λ = 468 nm
4.	Curing	>55°C (70°C)	Any temperature

(Contd.)

(Contd.)

S. No.	Considerations	Heat cured	Cold-self cured
5.	Curing time	Longer	Shorter
6.	Porosity	More	Less
7.	Dimensional accuracy	Less	Better and fits well
8.	Instruments and techniques	More complicated	Simpler
9.	Biological	Better	More residual MMA allergic
10.	Mechanical	Better	Poor—due to lower degree of polymerization
11.	Esthetics	Better	Poor, slow yellowing due to residual amines

Note on denture repair resins

These may be either heat cured or cold cured acrylic resins normally supplied as powder/liquid systems like denture base resins, but with finer particles. The parts of the broken denture are assembled on the cast and are joined by molten sticky wax, flasking, and dewaxing is done. The acrylic repair resin dough is packed cured by conventional method, and finished. Even though heat cured acrylics have better properties, it is not used, as repeated heating and cooling can cause warpage and misfit of the denture.

SHORT ESSAYS

3. Define dental cast. Write advantages and disadvantages of gypsum products as cast materials.

Dental casts are the exact hard duplicates of oral structures, including the associated soft tissues, used for preparing the wax patterns for dentures, or study models in orthodontic treatments. These are commonly prepared using type III dental stone (autoclaved/Hydrocal: $CaSO_4.\frac{1}{2}H_2O$. The powder is mixed with water, using proper w/p ratio (28–35%) and the cast is prepared by pouring the mix into the impression.

Setting reaction

When weighed amount of powder is added to measured volume of water:

$2\ CaSO_4.\frac{1}{2}\ H_2O + 3\ H_2O \rightarrow 2\ CaSO_4.2\ H_2O +$ heat (3900 cal/gm.mol).

The $CaSO_4.2H_2O$ formed sets into a hard mass

Advantages

- Adequate compressive strength (in 1 hr >26 MPa and dry strength (60–70 MPa)
- Good dimensional stability—NSE <0.2%.
- Controllable setting time and setting expansions (by HSE)
- Simple method and adequate shelf-life.

Disadvantages

- Very brittle and low fracture resistance.
- Hygroscopic powder and the cast also cannot be stored for long time.
- Inadequate abrasive resistance (surface hardeners should be used).

4. Condensation silicones *vs* addition silicones

These are two varieties of elastomeric impression materials having long chained coiled polymeric structures with limited cross-linking, exhibiting large visicoelastic and elastic recovery properties. Their consistencies are adjusted by the amount of filler (light—16%, regular—25%, heavy—36% and putty >50%).

Both are supplied in two paste systems of light, regular, heavy and putty consistencies. Condensation polysilicone base paste contains low molecular weight poly dimethyl siloxane with—OH-terminal group, colloidal silica fillers, plasticizers and tin octovate catalyst. Reactor paste has ethyl silicate, fillers and plasticizers. When these are mixed, ethyl silicate cross-links and ethyl alcohol byproduct is formed.

Addition polysilicone base paste contains low molecular weight poly dimethyl hydrogen siloxane with silane groups, colloidal silica fillers, plasticizers and chloroplatinic acid catalyst. Reactor paste has, low molecular weight poly dimethyl vinyl siloxane with vinyl, ($-CH = CH_2$), terminal group, fillers and plasticizers. On mixing addition polymerization reaction takes place with limited cross-linking, without byproduct.

Comparison of properties

Properties	Cond polysilicone	Add polysilicone
Elastic recovery	99.5%	99.93% (highest)
COTE thermal shrinkage	190 ppm/°C	190 ppm/°C (same)
Polymerization shrinkage	More	Less
Flow at 1 hr	0.09%	0.05% (lower)
Flexibility	4–9%	3.0% (lower)
Tear strength (regular)	3500 gm/cm	3500 gm/cm (same)
Hardness (LRHP)	Adequate (good)	Adequate (good)
Dimensional stability	Poorer—byproducts	Good

Additional polysilicone is preferred due to its higher dimensional stability, even though, the flexibility is lower. The monophase pseudoplastic material has more advantages as it can be used in simpler, single mix single impression technique. Evolving H_2 gas is absorbed by added Pt, or Pd dust. Cast pouring is to be delayed for 30 min for maximum elastic recovery. Tray adhesives should be used in both the cases.

Applications: To record very accurate impressions for the fabrications of inlays, onlays, crowns and bridges, partial and complete dentures.

5. Modifications of GIC

Glass ionomer cements are recent popular biocompatible, anticariogenic, chemically bonding to tooth, anterior restorative materials, supplied as powder/liquid systems in many types for different uses.

These are modified to overcome some of their drawbacks such as, inadequate early strengths, slow setting actions, moisture sensitivity, brittleness, etc.

(1) Metal modified GICs have two varieties

Miracle-mix of Dr. Siemen: Spherical silver amalgam alloy powder is mixed with type 2 GIC powder. Strength is increased to about 150–200 MPa but it became more opaque—can be used for core-building.

Glass cermet cement of Dr. Macleans': Silver or gold powder in high density is sintered along with glass ingredients (ceramic + metal). Strength increased to about 200 MPa, but esthetics decreased.

Uses: Core build-up materials, liners under composite resins.

(2) Resin modified GIC (other names: Hybrid ionomer, compomer, resinomer, vitremer, direct dual- or tri-cure ionomers, etc.)

Powder contains ion-leachable silica, alumina glasses, fluorides, resin matrix (BISGMA), coupling agents (organo vinyl silanes), initiators (dimethyl-p-toluidine for chemical, or camphorquinone for light activation). Liquid is aqueous solution of polyacrylic acid with modified methyl methacrylate and HEMA (hydroxyethyl methacrylate, and dimethyl amino-ethyl methacrylate.

- Di-cure GIC sets by acid–base and polymerization reactions.
- Tri-cure GIC sets by acid-base, polymerization and light curing reactions. This includes photoreactive camphorquinones and has shorter setting time as desired and also dentist's command setting properties.

Properties

- Anticariogenic, biocompatible, chemically adhesive, lower solubility, mild pulpal response, etc.
- Lower mechanical properties (lower compressive strength = 105 MPa, tensile strength = 20 MPa, surface hardness = 40 KHN), limits its uses to liners, luting, pit and fissure sealants, cement bases, etc. The compomers are sometimes dispensed in capsules.

Uses: Core build-up materials, liners under composite resins, cement bases, pit and fissure sealants.

6. Properties of 18-8 stainless steel

Compositions

Austenitic (fcc) 18-8 stainless steel contains chromium = 18% for passivation, nickel = 8% for depressing martensitic formation temperatures, carbon = 0.15% (<0.2%) for strengthening, manganese = 2%, and iron = balance.

Properties

Corrosion

- *Passivation:* Chromium >11.5%, present in 18–8 stainless steel combines with atmospheric oxygen and forms an impervious chromic oxide layer on the surface and at grain boundaries, preventing further entry of oxygen and corrosion.
- *Sensitization:* Loss of corrosion resistance, when it is heated above 350°C. As the temperature rises the carbon atoms diffuse to the grain boundaries and the surfaces, and combine with chromium to form $(CrFe)_4C$. This reduces the number of chromium atoms on the surface and hence, decreases the corrosion resistance. *Weld-decay* at the welded parts of stainless steel articles and also at the soldered joints are due to this. Hence, low-fusing solders are to be used and the procedures are to be done very quickly.
- *Stabilization:* Addition of **niobium or titanium with tantalum about six times** carbon, arrests temporarily the diffusion of carbon atoms at high temperatures and prevents sensitization.

Biocompatibilities of low carbon stainless steels are good and hence are used for dental and orthopedic implants.

Mechanical properties

- *Highly ductile and malleable:* Thin wires for orthodontic passive appliances, thin sheets of <1/20th mm thickness tried for denture bases, are examples. Density is about 8.3 gm/cc.
- *Good mechanical properties*: High YS = 1,760 MPa, high UTS = 2,100 MPa. High abrasive resistance (SH = 250–350 KHN), high MOE = 200,000 MPa. Large % elongation

= 35%, etc. are suited for passive orthodontic appliances, i.e. to resist undesired movements of teeth.

Thermal properties: Good conductor of heat and electricity. High fusion temperature ranges = 1240°–1260°C.

Applications

- *Orthodontia:* Wires (passive appliances), brackets, etc.
- *Dental clinical instruments:* Burs, carvers, excavators, etc., equipment.
- Dental implants, orthopedic implants, bone-plates, hip joints, rods, nuts, bolts, etc.
- Household utensils, machine parts—equipment in industries, machine parts, etc.

Note: Select short answers for corrosion, passivation, stabilization and weld decay of 18-8 stainless steel.

7. Abrasive agents

Abrasion is a method of removing unwanted materials from the surface of an article and obtaining even surface, by moving hard abrasive particles, i.e. wearing by moving the abrasive agents over the surface and cutting them.

The abrasive agents should have:

- High attrition resistance and higher surface hardness than the work.
- Very hard, brittle, and should fracture easily, forming large number of irregular new sharp-edged particles for abrasion.

Common abrasive agents are diamond particles (having highest SH >5000 KHN or even >10,000 KHN). Carbides (SH = 2,500 KHN), Alumina-emery (SH = 2,000 KHN). Quartz or sand = SH >800 KHN), metal oxides, etc. These are powdered into fine particles of different grit sizes (40, 60, 80, —180, etc.).

These are used as:

- Unbonded abrasives like coarse or finer alumina, sand powders, metal oxides ZnO, Fe_2O_3, ZrO, etc. used directly (e.g. sand blasting, air abrasions, bicarbonate—mild abrasives of dentifrices, etc.)
- *Coated abrasives:* Abrasive powders, sand, emery, etc are coated on papers, plastic sheets or metal strips.

- *Bonded abrasives:* The abrasive powders are bonded to rotating shafts of abrasive tools—diamond points or discs, carbide burs, stones, etc. The bonding is done by sintering, vitreous, resinoid, rubber, etc techniques.

Abrasion is done by moving the abrasive tools *unidirectionally*, on the work surface without applying much pressure (since it is difficult to remove deep scratches). The grit size should be selected in the descending order of particle sizes.

The efficiency of abrasion depends on
- The surface hardness of abrasives and work surface.
- Speed of abrasion and load applied.
- Attrition resistance and brittleness of abrasive agents, etc.

[Optional-polishing agents are very fine powder particles of abrasives (like diamond pastes-for metal polishing, ZrO, Fe_2O_3—rouge, pumice, etc. for metals and cement restorations, pumice, and French chalk for acrylics, etc.) of sizes <10 microns, supplied as 0, 00, 000, or F, FF, FFF grits. Their slurries in water, or glycerin with cotton or rotating buffs are pressed and moved in multidirections after abrasion, Minimum material is removed, microcrystalline or Beilby layer is formed and glossy smooth surface is obtained].

8. Flow and viscosity of dental materials

Flow is the property of amorphous and viscoelastic materials undergoing time-dependent deformations by their own weight or under external deforming forces. This time-dependent deformations, of crystalline materials such as silver amalgam is known as creep, which is static or dynamic, under repeated loadings. Acrylic dentures also undergo creep. Often, the terms—creep and flow are confused and used for both. Flows or creeps increase with temperatures.

Measurements
- Flow of impression compound is measured by the % deformations taking place by a disc of 10 mm diameter and 6 mm height under a load of 2.5 kg for 10 mt at 37°C and 46°C temperatures. For type 1, these should be <6% and >85%. Flow of hydrocolloids and elastomers are

measured by standard methods. Higher flow and elastic recoveries are required for accurate impressions.

- Creep of silver amalgam is measured by preparing acylindrical sample of height: 8 mm and diameter: 4 mm, maintaining at 37°C for 7 days and then applying a load of 36 newtons. The % deformations taking place between the ends of 1 hr and 4 hr, is creep. ADA specification is < 2%. Single composition high copper amalgam has least creep about 0.05–0.1%. Creep should be minimum to avoid marginal fractures and ditching of restorations.

- *Viscosity* is the resistance of liquids (fluids) for the deformations. *It is measured by the force acting between two adjacent layers of unit area of a liquid maintaining unit velocity gradient, at stream-lined motion. This has the unit stress/strain rate.* This is expressed in MPa-second or Poise (or centi-Poise). Liquids do not have elastic recovery properties. When stressed, they undergo time dependent permanent deformations or have strain rates. For example, viscosity of water at 20°C is 1 cP. For elastomers, these vary according to their consistencies— 60,000 to 450,000 cP and temperatures. The viscosity decreases as temperature, rises.

- The viscosity refers to consistencies of dental materials. The impression material mixes of thinner consistencies have better flow and produce more accurate reproduction of finer details of oral structures (e.g. ZnOE, light-body elastomers, and agar-agar). The consistencies of restorative and luting cements are also equally important.

- The viscosity or thinness decreases when higher shearing forces are applied in case of pseudoplastic materials. (plaster mix, $ZnPO_4$, cement mix, monophase (single consistency) elastomers.

In all cases of setting materials, the consistencies are controlled by fillers and increases rapidly with time and also temperatures. Consistencies are measured by placing 0.5 ml of standard mix in-between two glass plates under definite loads for 10 min or so. Diameters of the material discs formed are referred as consistencies (e.g. ZnOE, impression mixes, ZnOE, $ZnPO_4$, luting, and base cements).

9. Fillers and resin matrix in dental composites

Composite resins are three-dimensional structures of two or more chemically different materials insoluble in each other, with an interface material, chemically binding them together to obtain desired superior properties. These are fillers, resin matrix and keying or coupling agents.

Fillers are hard chemically inert material particles of very small sizes in the form of powders, beads, cylinders, etc. Functions of fillers in composite resins are to increase strength, abrasive resistance and esthetics, reduce thermal shrinkages (COTE), controls viscosity, workability, radio-opacity and reduces water absorption.

- *The inorganic fillers* are of quartz, pyrolytic silica, aluminum silicate, lithium–aluminum silicate (β-eucreptite), borosilicate or barium glasses. These are treated with vinyl silane coupling agents to chemically bond with the resin matrix to enhance the strengths. According to filler particle sizes there are: Large, small, micro, nano, hybrid (mixtures of micro and small: fillers) composite resins.
- *Organic fillers* are prepared by mixing the coupling agent-silane-treated colloidal silica with monomers and chloroform at slightly higher temperature, heat curing with benzoyl peroxide initiator and then powdering. This inorganic fillers control viscosity and increases the filler load.

Resin matrix

- High molecular weight resin matrix, bisphenol glycidyl methacrylate (BISGMA), known as Bowen's resin (1960), undergoes free radical addition polymerization, forming highly cross-linked rigid resin matrix while setting. This can be polymerized by chemical initiators (benzoyl peroxide–dimethyl-p-toluidine), ultraviolet rays ($\lambda = 350$ nm) or visible light ($\lambda = 468$ nm). But this is very highly viscous monomer. Low molecular weight thinner monomers, triethylene glycol dimethacrylate (TEGDMA) is usually mixed with BISGMA in 1:3 ratio. The composite resins of different varieties are used for anterior and posterior restorations, pit and fissure sealants, etc.

10. Castable ceramics

Castable ceramics were developed to avail the best esthetic properties for restorations and introduced by Dentsply International Corning (DICOR) glass company. A hard ceramic die is first prepared. Thick wax pattern with short sprue is prepared and is divested in phosphate bonded divestment material, and dewaxed. The glass pellets are melted in a ceramic crucible and casting is done using centrifugal casting machine. The cast is recovered.

Ceramming is conducted, by embedding this clear transparent cast glass in a protective investment and maintained at about 800°C for about 10–12 hr. *Devitrification*, in the middle of the articles, causes mica-like crystals of higher refractive index. This contributes better esthetics: Chameleon effect. Later cementation is done.

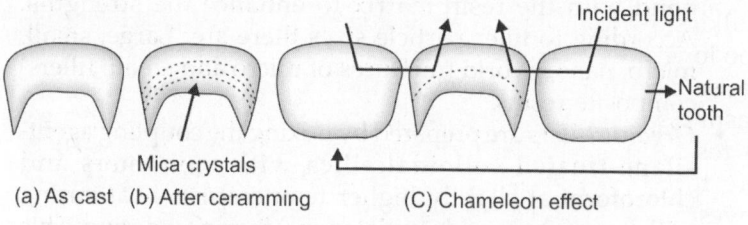

(a) As cast (b) After ceramming   (C) Chameleon effect

This DICOR is not used nowadays since:

- It is brittle and has low tensile strength and fractures easily.
- These thick restorations require removal of more, healthier tooth materials.

Modifications

- Injection moulding technique: The leucite containing ceramic pellets are softened or fused at about 1080°C and injected instead of casting in centrifugal casting machine, or,
- The ceramic powder is blended in a resin, softened at about 250°C and injected into the mould at high pressure.
- The ceramic ingots are softened by heating, and then hot-pressed into the mold for about 45 min.

- These have better flexure strength, and fitting but poor esthetics than metal ceramics. All these can be cerammed to have better esthetics. But these methods are more complicated.

SHORT ANSWERS

11. Sprue former

Sprue is a channel or ingate to the mould of the wax pattern in the invested casting ring to drain out the molten wax and later to allow the molten alloy liquid to enter and completely fill the mould.

It is made up of wax ropes of thickness, 1.3–2.6 mm (slightly thicker than the thickest part of wax pattern) and of length, to position the wax pattern in the middle of investing casting ring. Spruing is done directly to single pattern or indirectly to more patterns for single casting, with a drop of molten wax at the bulkiest part, inclined at 45° to the occlusal plane. Too thin or too long sprue cause pre-solidification of alloy liquid in it and cause incomplete castings. Too thick or short sprues increase casting speed, abrade investment and result in rough surface. A reservoir is created near the wax pattern. Fine vent sprues are to be fitted in case of nonporous phosphate bonded investments (Draw diagram—Colour Plate 37, Fig. 62).

12. Tray adhesives

Many impression materials like hydrocolloids and elastomers do not bond to the metal or acrylic trays and detachment of impression cause distortions. Mechanical bonding of hydrocolloid impressions is done in the perforated trays by the set tag formed materials.

Tray adhesives of different types are applied on the tray surfaces before loading the mixed elastomeric impression material. For polysulphides butyl rubber or styrene dissolved in chloroform or ketones can be used. Poly dimethyl siloxane or ethyl silicates are used in case of polysilicones.

13. Microleakage

One main purpose of the restoration of the missing part of the tooth is to protect the delicate pulp from the external irritants entering and damaging it. But even after the restorations, the irritant fluids may enter, if the marginal gaps are created. This is known as marginal or microleakage, which results in failure of the restoration.

Causes for microleakages

- No chemical bonding of restoratives to tooth.
- Setting contraction.
- Marginal dissolution or disintegration.
- Dissimilar COTEs of restorative and tooth. When hot or cold foods/beverages are taken marginal percolation takes place.

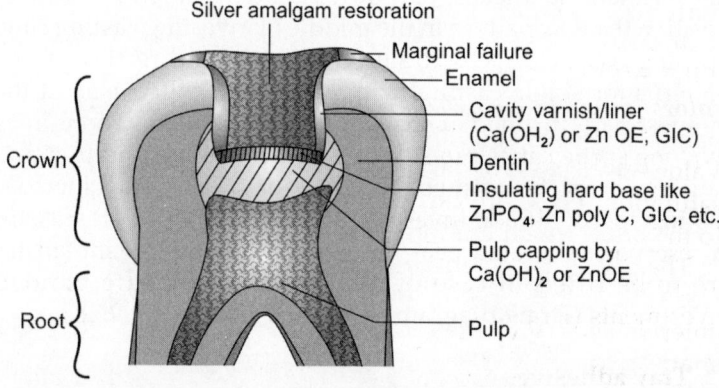

Microleakage can be minimized by choosing proper material, correct method of restoration and applying cavity varnishes (thin coating of natural gums, rosins or synthetic resins dissolved in organic solvents—acetone, chloroform or ethers).

14. Gutta-percha

This is naturally occurring polymeric material, chemically known as, transisomer of polyisoprene, obtained from latex or similar rubbers. It is supplied as rods of 3 mm diameter—10 cm lengths or narrow cones of certain dimensions in different colors.

Compositions: Gutta-percha, ZnO, barium sulphate, waxes, etc.

On warming and cooling, it undergoes transitions from β gutta-percha 50°C ↔ α gutta-percha 56–62°C ↔ γ phases with dimensional changes.

Uses: Gutta-percha is mainly used for root canal sealing, by warm-up method-softening and plugging into the root canal, or the plugger itself can be warmed earlier. Other techniques are: Cold up, semi dissolved condition (chloro-percha or euco-percha), injecting methods, etc. Gutta-percha is inert dimensionally stable and has good adapting properties. Sometimes it is also used *for functional impressions of cleft palate cases.*

15. Significance of color in dentistry

Esthetic consideration of restorative materials for exact color-matching is of prime concern for selection of anterior restoratives. Combinations of different *primary colors* in different proportions *(red, green, and blue)* produce *secondary colors (magenta, cyan and yellow) which produce* various color parameters corresponding to: Hue—dominant wavelengths, Value—brightness or darkness of the surface, and chroma-color saturation. These are carried by the rod and cone nerve ends to the brain which interprets accordingly.

The color parameters are measured by using Munsel's color tree or spectroscopic methods. The manufacturers prepare anterior restorative materials of different shades and provide shade guide tabs for visible comparison method of color matching.

Since the structures of dentin and enamel are anisotropic, i.e. refractive indices of dentin and enamels, H,V,C, values vary from point to point, at different directions and for different wavelengths, ideal materials cannot be manufactured or perfect color matching cannot be achieved.

2. RAJIV GANDHI UNIVERSITY OF HEALTH SCIENCES
II Year BDS Degree Examination, December 2015
DENTAL MATERIALS (RS-3)
QP CODE: 1185

LONG ESSAYS 2 × 10 = 20 marks

1. Classify dental amalgam alloys and describe the steps in manipulation of high copper amalgam alloys.

2. Describe in detail about abrasive and polishing agents.

SHORT ESSAYS 8 × 5 = 40 marks

3. Distortion and remedies of inlay waxes.

4. Adverse effect of dental materials.

5. Metal ceramic bonding.

6. Types of glass ionomer cements.

7. Eutectic and peritectic alloys.

8. Components of composite resin.

9. Firing procedure in dental ceramics.

10. Explain different types of denture base resin in brief.

SHORT ANSWERS 5 × 2 = 10 marks

11. Eame's technique

12. Elastic limit

13. Super-cooled liquids

14. Spherulites

15. Die spacers

Answers

LONG ESSAYS

1. Classify dental amalgam alloys and describe the steps in manipulation of high copper amalgam alloys.

Dental amalgam or silver amalgam is an alloy of mercury with an alloy of silver, tin and copper. It was popular direct filling posterior restorative material.

After GV Black's first formulation (1890), several types of these silver–tin, copper, etc., alloys came into use to overcome the drawbacks.

These are classified for selecting quickly most suitable material required to the clinical treatments, according to

1. **Compositions**
   - Low copper alloy (Cu <6%)
   - High copper alloy (Cu >13%)—admix
   - High copper alloy (Cu >13%)—single composition
   - Zinc containing or non-zinc alloys
   - Gallium alloy

2. **Particle shapes**
   - Irregular lathe-cut
   - Spherical silver–copper alloys
   - Admix or disperse (mixture of irregular lathe-cut and silver–copper eutectic spherical alloys)

3. **Particle size**
   - Microcut <35 microns
   - Fine cut >35 microns

4. **Dispensing methods**
   - Powder—liquid (mercury) system
   - Powder—pellet and liquid mercury
   - Pre-proportioned, disposable capsules

5. **Special treatments**
   - Aged alloys
   - Acid washed
   - Pre-amalgamated alloys

Manipulation steps

Criteria for selection of alloys: High 1 hour and final strengths, good corrosion resistance, least creep and dimensional changes.

Selection: High copper single composition, fine particle size, aged or heat treated, zinc-free alloys. *Mercury should be triple-distilled pure and arsenic-free.*

Proportioning: Suitable mercury alloy ratio is taken, depending on the compositions. For earlier increasing dryness technique Hg/alloy ratio was 50–54% by wt for low copper lathe-cut alloys, about 48–50% by wt. for single composition high copper alloys, and for **Eame's minimal mercury technique** Hg/alloy ratio is **1:1** by weight. Volume dispensers or amalgamators are used.

Trituration methods

Mercury cannot easily wet the alloy powder due to its large surface tension (460 dynes/cm), high angle of contact (135°) and metal oxide layers. When the powder is mixed with mercury they do not react. Trituration is required to remove oxide layers and produce reaction.

Hand trituration: The proportioned mercury and alloy powders are placed in a clean glass mortar. The glass pestle is held *in palm or fist grip* and the trituration is done to obtain a homogeneous thick consistency. *For hand trituration (mixing)* time is about *45 to 60 seconds*. If the powder taken is more or not mixed adequately, many *dark spots* can be observed. Correct mix has shining, thick, paste-like consistency. If too much mercury is added, the mix becomes very thin and shining, like mercury. Using squeeze cloth, excess mercury is removed. *Hand mulling* by rubbing the mix in the palm by a finger is done to get *homogeneous mix*. Then it is condensed into cavity in increments by applying large force about *1.5–1.7 kg*.

Mechanical trituration

The proportioned mercury and alloy powders are taken in air tight plastic capsule. It is then vibrated vigorously for about 20–30 seconds by an electrical vibrator. Sometimes a small cylindrical plastic rod kept inside the capsule, act as pestle. The capsule is opened after a short time (for mercury vapor to settle). The plastic rod is removed and the closed capsule is again quickly vibrated. This *mechanical mulling forms* uniform consistency, which can be rolled into a sphere.

Sometimes special *disposable capsules* containing pre-proportioned mercury and alloy powder in separate compartments are supplied. This is directly vibrated.

Amalgamator used in clinics, has mercury and powder in separate compartments. By turning a knob, proportioned volumes get collected in a special capsule which is violently vibrated (for 25 to 30 sec). Speed and time of vibration are controlled by a rheostat and timer. *This gives a standard reproducible mix.* If required excess mercury is squeezed out, mulling is done and condensed into the cavity.

- This mix is then carried to the cavity floor (already laid with a cement base) and condensed by applying about 1.6 kg force uniformly.
- Excess mercury is removed leaving a little behind for bonding the next increment. Next increments are condensed one after the other, each time leaving the surface more and more dry, until the cavity is slightly overfilled for carving. This *increasing dryness technique* is more complicated.
- In Eame's *technique mercury/alloy ratio is 1:1 by wt and excess of mercury is not removed.* Initial carving can be done after half an hour.
- Final polishing and burnishing are delayed for 24 hours for low copper alloys. High copper amalgam restoration can be finished *in single sitting as it has adequate high one-hour strength, 270 MPa.*

Precautions

- Moisture contamination during condensation cause delayed expansion of Zn containing alloys and should be avoided by using rubber dams.
- Homogeneous condensation is a must, otherwise thinner-mercury rich portions get moved to the margins. This will cause further reaction and cause mercuroscopic expansion and ditching of restoration.
- *Overtrituration* produces greater amounts of weaker reaction products, gamma one and gamma 2 or neta phases and the strength decreases, the dimensional changes and creep become greater.

- *Undertrituration* causes improper wetting of powder with mercury and inhomogeneous mix. Hence, it decreases strength, and cannot be condensed properly.

2. Describe in detail about abrasive and polishing agents

Abrasive agents are powders of hard materials with irregular particles having sharp edges. For example, diamond powder, carbides, aluminum oxides, sand, pumice, etc. These are used to cut and remove the unwanted materials from the surface of the work to get desired shape and sizes, in the finishing steps.

1. **Bonded abrasives:** These abrasives are bonded to rotating discs, grinding wheels and shafts (e.g. diamond points, carbide burs, grinding stones, discs, etc.).
2. **Coated abrasives:** These particles are coated on plastic cloth, or paper or strips. For example, emery, sand papers, metal oxide coated strips. These are numbered accordingly to grit size, 40, 60, 80, 100, 120, ... 600, etc.
3. **Unbonded abrasive powder:** Coarse or fine alumina or sand powders used directly in sand blasting technique, dentifrice, air abrasion techniques, etc.

Some abrasives are diamond, carbides of boron, tungsten or silicones, oxides of aluminum, iron, zirconium or silicones (some oxide ores are pumice, kieselgur, etc.)

Mild abrasives like calcium or sodium bicarbonates are used in dentifrices. Lavigated alumina, zirconium oxide or silica is used in prophy-pastes.

Abrasive actions: These abrasive agents are applied on the surface without applying much pressure and moved in a *single direction*. This process removes the unwanted material on the surface which has been properly shaped by cutting instruments, like burs. Proper abrasive agents are first selected. It is used successively, from coarse to fine (smaller grit size) until a smooth regular surface is obtained.

Polishing agents

These are **very fine hard particles**, of sizes <10 microns like diamond, carbides, alumina, sand, metal oxides, pumice, French chalk, etc. denoted as 0, 00, 000, or F, FF, FFF. These are mixed with glycerine or water to form *thick slurry* and applied on the surface through cotton (or rotating cotton, felt or silk buffs) in *multidirections. During polishing, minimal or no material is removed.* This forms a *microcrystalline or Beilby layer,* which is very *smooth and glossy.* For polishing metallic appliances, silver amalgam, composite resins, fine powders of pumice, kieselgur, Tripoli, etc. can be used by forming slurry.

- Finishing of acrylic denture is done by first abrading with sand papers of decreasing grit size and then polishing by pumice and finally with French chalk—slurries or rouge.
- Smooth surfaces of ceramic restorations are obtained by glazing. Glaze or unfilled composites are used for finishing composite resin restorations. Electropolishing is done for PBM alloy appliances.
- Well polished (finished) restorations do not collect food debris or irritate the opposing tissues. These have better esthetics, higher corrosion resistance and hygienic.

SHORT ESSAYS   8 × 5 = 40 marks

3. Distortion and remedies of inlay waxes

Inlay pattern waxes contain thermoplastic materials like paraffin waxbees' wax, carnauba wax, gum-dammar, synthetic resins, etc. having high COTE (300–700 ppm/°C), and very low thermal conductivities.

- Type 1: Medium wax is used for direct pattern on the prepared tooth.
- Type 2: Soft wax is used to prepare wax pattern indirectly outside the mouth, i.e. on the die of tooth.

During preparation of wax pattern, the molecules are displaced causing internal stresses. While cooling, due to low thermal conductivity and large thermal contractions, the outer part solidifies first and inside later. This also causes internal stresses. *Relaxation of these internal stresses cause distortion of wax patterns. Distortion and shrinkages cause misfit.*

Precautions (methods) for minimizing distortion

- Select the proper type of waxes as specified by ADA.
- Soften the wax uniformly.
- Place the softened or molten increments quickly to bond with earlier increment.

- After the overfilled pattern hardens, carefully do the carving without pulling away from the margins.
- Remove the pattern very carefully (a drop of oil or lubricant applied on the prepared cavity or die, facilitates this).
- Invest the pattern immediately without delay or it can be stored in cold water (in a refrigerator for a short time).

4. Adverse effect of dental materials

Many materials are used in the oral cavity, temporarily or permanently in contact with soft and hard tissues and sometimes as implants. These should be biocompatible and should not produce any adverse effects.

- Acidic cements may cause pulpal irritation.
- Polymeric material (PMMA—denture base) may contain unreacted monomer, which cause allergies.
- Mercury used in dental amalgam may be toxic, if proper precautions are not taken.
- Dust from alginate impression material may cause *silicosis* if inhaled frequently for long time.
- Some casting alloys such as nickel causes nickel toxicity.
- Beryllium can cause *berylliosis*, if the *berillium (Be) dust or vapor inhaled* during grinding of cast restorations or during manufacturing, may affect the lungs, skin, eyes or blood and the affects can occur immediately or after long-term exposure.
- Uranium is sometimes added to dental porcelain composition, can cause adverse reactions and should be handled properly.
- Heavy metals such as lead and tin are used in elastomeric impression materials should be handled with proper care, direct contact with soft tissues can lead to adverse reactions.
- Eugenol in impression paste can cause burning sensation in some patients.
- Dressing materials used in periodontal treatments may contain asbestos fibers which can lead to local reactions in the oral cavity.

Auxiliary materials (laboratory materials), can contain some hazardous materials such as cyanide solution for electroplating, vapors from low fusing metal dies, siliceous particles from impression materials and abrasives (silicosis), fluxes containing fluoride, asbestos dust, etc. All the above materials may lead to adverse reactions, and should be handled carefully.

Causes and symptoms

Coughing, shortness of breath and weight loss that begin abruptly can be a symptom of acute *berylliosis.* This condition is caused by beryllium air pollution that inflames the lungs making them rigid, it can affect the eyes and skin as well. People who have acute berylliosis are usually very ill, most recover, but some die of the disease.

Biocompatibility tests are required to take suitable precautions, and to avoid such materials.

5. Metal ceramic bonding

Metal ceramic appliances are made to incorporate the desired strength of metals and esthetics of ceramics. Due to high surface tension (about 365 dynes / cm), and large angle of contact (about 135°), ceramic liquid cannot wet metal surface and bond with it. Hence, following methods are used for metal ceramic bonding.

1. *Mechanical bonding:* The bonding surface of the cast metal is made rough by using diamond or carbide burs and discs, or sand blasting.
2. *Thermal mismatching the COTE by 0.5 ppm/°C.* This is done by adding Pd, Pt, etc. to the alloys to reduce COTE down to 13.5 to 14 ppm/°C and adding devitrifiers to ceramics or using leucite which increases COTE of ceramics to about 13–13.5 ppm/°C.
3. *Chemical bonding:* This is achieved by bonding of ceramics through oxygen of the *tin oxide layer* formed on the metal surface.

Methods

After the HN or N alloys metallic portion cast is finished, a thin layer of pure gold is deposited by electrolysis, and then a flash deposition of tin is electrodeposited over it. *Degassing* is done by heating this to about 900°C for a few minutes. Any gas included will be driven out and a thin *tin oxide layer* is formed on its surface. This chemically *bonds* it with ceramics. It is cooled, and layers of different ceramics (dentin, cervical,

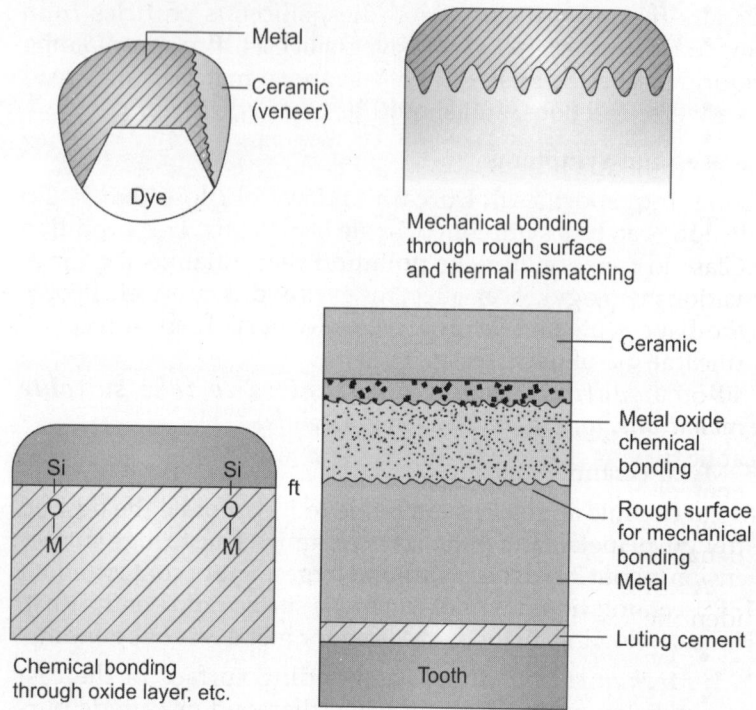

color frits, enamel, etc,) are applied and fired one after the other, which bond by thermal mismatching. The gold color gives a vital esthetics.

In case of PBM alloy castings, after finishing, surface is sand blasted, i.e. roughened, for mechanical bonding. This is degassed and then applied with opaquer slurry and fired. This is to mask the nonvital-white color reflections from the surface. The chemical bonding takes place through the oxide layer of chromium, etc. This is repeated successively with increment layers of dentin porcelain, enamel porcelain, color frits and finally glazed.

Metal ceramic bond failures

Labelled diagram

The metal or ceramic appliances contain strong and tough alloys bonded with hard brittle ceramic through metal oxide layer. Hence, bond failures can take place under tensile stresses at:

- Metal and metal oxide interface, due to poor bonding.
- Within the metal oxide layer, due to thicker oxide layer which is weaker than metal or ceramic.
- Metal oxide–ceramic junction, due to weak bonding.
- Failure also can take place at the metal or ceramic regions, if these are weaker than the bond strength.

6. Types of glass ionomer cements

Glass ionomer cements (GICs) are the materials of choice for various types of anterior and other types of restorations. GICs are dispensed as fine glass powders or nanoparticles containing silica, alumina, fluorides of Ca, Na, K, etc. and liquid containing 40–50% of aqueous solutions of polyacrylic acid, itaconic acid, maleic acids, etc. GICs have many desirable properties such as anticariogenic, biocompatibility, chemically bonding to tooth enamel and dentin, good esthetics, etc. Due to these attractive properties, many types have been prepared and dispensed usually as powder liquid systems.

According to applications, the following types have been identified:

- Type I: Luting
- Type II: Restoration
- Type III: Cavity liners, cement bases
- Type IV: Fissure sealant
- Type V: Orthodontic cement
- Type VI: Core build up
- Fuji VII: *The world's first fluoride non-resin containing auto-cure GIC.*
- Fuji VIII and Fuji IX: *Atraumatic restorative* (ART) materials (also referred as *gediatric* or pediatric materials)

Some of the drawbacks of GICs are, poor strength, low fracture resistance, low abrasion resistance (inadequate for posterior restorations), as well as slow setting, many modifications are used for different applications. Metal modified varieties of GICs are ***miracle-mix and cermets.*** Resin modified GICs are ***resinomers, compomers, dual-cured*** (by acid–base and polymerizing actions), tri cured (by light curing, acid–base and polymerizing actions).

7. Eutectic and peritectic alloys

Eutectic alloys have partially soluble metals, having a *single lowest* solidification or melting temperature for a definite compositional ratio. For example, silver and copper have their melting temperatures, 961°C and 1083°C respectively and both have FCC lattices. **Eutectic alloy formed has *silver = 72% and copper = 28%*.** This has single, lowest melting temperature 779°C. The maximum solubility of copper in silver 8.8% and that of silver in copper is 8%, at this eutectic temperature.

Eutectic phase

During enmasse solidification at 779°C, *alternate layers of copper in silver, α and silver in copper, β solid solutions are formed.*

Liquid → α (alpha) solid solution + β (beta) solid solution at eutectic, lowest temperature in alternate layer.

This eutectic phase has high slip resistance, i.e. high strength and brittleness. This phase, therefore, cannot be heat hardened or softened.

Hypoeutectic phase: This has primary α (*alpha*) crystals embedded in eutectic phase, when copper percentage is between 8.8% and 28%. This phase is still more brittle.

Hypereutectic phase: This has primary β (beta) crystals (Ag in Cu), crystals embedded in eutectic phase, when the percentage of copper is between 28% and 92%. This also has greater brittleness and strength than eutectic phase.

Applications

Admixed high copper silver amalgam alloys powder contain 1 part of silver-copper eutectic alloy; spherical particles, mixed with 2 parts of low copper lathe-cut alloys. Eutectic phase is supposed to act *as filler.*

Grain refinement is done by the lower eutectic temperature formed by adding some trace elements like Ir, Ru, W, etc. to HN, N or PBM casting alloys.

Peritectic (transformations) alloys

Peritectic means going around. When an alloy (e.g. Pt–Ag) of particular composition solidifies, new phase is formed by the atoms in the liquid condition going around and form new phase. The peritectic transformation can be represented as β (solid solution) + alloy liquid → γ solid solution phase.

Example: During the solidification of silver-tin alloy having 27% tin, the primary disordered beta solid solution in the alloy liquid, changes to ordered gama intermetallic phase (Ag_3Sn) by the diffusion of tin atoms as represented. If the liquid is solidified quickly, less gamma phase forms around beta crystals.

Ratio of gamma and beta phases can, hence be, controlled by the rate of solidification and cooling. This helps to control the amalgamation reaction rate, working and setting times.

[*Note:* When feldspathic porcelain is heated, *incongruent melting* takes place forming leaucite solid and liquid phases, i.e. reverse of peritectic changes.]

8. Components of composite resin

Composite resin can be defined as a three-dimensional polymeric structure of two or more chemically different substances, insoluble in each other and another chemical (coupling or keying agent) acting as an interface combining them together.

For example, the dental composite resins contain resin matrix and silica type fillers, coupled together by a coupling agent. This also contains initiators and activators (chemical, ultraviolet or visible light) along with opacifiers, shades, etc.

Compositions

Organic resin matrix

This is usually high molecular weight monomer of bis-phenolglycidyldimethacrylate (Bowen's resin) or BisGMA with or without OH group or urethane dimethacrylate, etc. These are very viscous and form highly cross-linked, hard structures. Sometimes, diluents like low mol wt monomer, dimethacrylates are added.

Fillers: *The fillers are added to increase the strength, abrasive resistance, transparency. These decrease the polymerization shrinkage and coefficient of thermal expansion.*

Inorganic fillers such as ground quartz, *precipitated pyrolytic silica,* aluminum silicate, lithium–aluminum silicate, borosilicate, barium glasses, etc., of different particle sizes varying from nanometer size to 8–12 microns, are used. Accordingly there are large particles (1–8 micron), small particles (1–5 µm), microsize (0.05–0.1), hybrid types (large particle, midifiller and minifiller), nanocomposites (<10 nm = 0.01 nm) are used.

Organic fillers

Since conventional composite resins containing large sized very hard filler particle cannot be polished, micro-sized fillers (0.04–0.06 µm) are used. To increase the filler loading and improve mechanical properties, *organic fillers* are used. First the colloidal silica particles of 0.04–0.06 µm are treated with coupling agents (vinyl silane), mixed with resin matrix, polymerized and broken into fine particles. These organic fillers are used in microfilled (polishable), flowable and glaze composites resins.

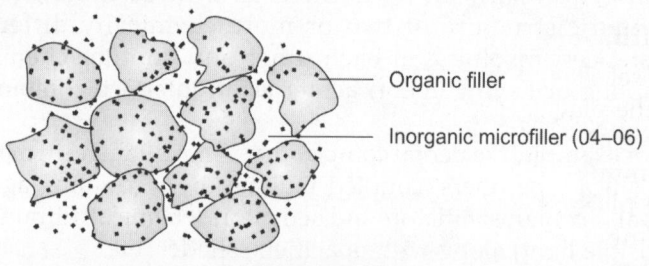

Organic filler

Inorganic microfiller (04–06)

Organic fillers

Coupling agents: These fillers are treated with vinyl silane, or γ **(gamma)-**methacryloxypropyl trimethoxysilanes, which can *chemically bond the silica and resin matrix. Coupling agents increase strength, acts as stress absorber and decrease polymerization shrinkage, and thermal expansion.*

Initiators and activators

1. *In chemically* or self cured material, N-N dimethyl para-toluidine is the activator and benzoyl peroxide is initiator.
2. *In ultraviolet* cured resins, *ultraviolet light of wavelength about 360 nm is activator and benzoin methyl ether is the initiator.*

3. *In visible light* cure systems (VLC), *light of wavelength 468 nm (or 460–480 nm) is the activator, camphoroquinone is the initiator with a tertiary amine (dimethyl amino-ethyl methacrylate) as accelerator.*

4. *Polymerization inhibitors,* like butylated hydroxyl toluene (BHT) is added to delay the polymerization to provide *adequate working time* and also long storage life.

5. *Color pigments,* TiO, Al_2O_3, BaO, etc. are added to provide a suitable shade and opacity to X-rays.

6. *UV absorbers or stabilizers, e.g. 2 hydroxy-4-methoxy benzoquinone.*

[*Note:* Many varieties of VLC composite resins are used for restorations (anterior, posterior), pit and fissure sealants, veneers, etc. Since it lacks chemical bonding and anticariogenic properties, it is modified with GIC—resinomers, compomers, etc.]

9. Firing procedure in dental ceramics

The selected ceramic slurry is applied and carefully condensed on the platinum foil adapted die and placed on the fire-clay-tray. This is placed on the platform near the open window of the muffle chamber, pre-heated to 650°C for 5 min for drying. The platform is raised and the article is held inside muffle chamber for 5 minutes. The remaining water is slowly converted into steam and comes out. The door of the muffle chamber is then closed. It is evacuated (by connecting it to a vacuum pump), immediately, in the case of vacuum firing technique, or filled with diffusible gases like H_2. or He, for reducing porosity. The temperature is gradually raised to about 950°C, i.e. firing temperature, in about 5 min (at the rate of 1°C per second). The article is kept at that temperature for a short time for the completion of the firing stages.

Stages of firing

- **Low bisque stage:** As the temperature gradually rises, the surface particles begin to soften and the lose particles first begin to join. There is no volume shrinkage and no cohesion. Firing is stopped in case of glass infiltrated core ceramics technique.

- **Medium bisque stage:** On further heating, more softening of particles takes place which begin to melt. There is better cohesion and slight volume shrinkage.
- **High bisque stage:** Further heating causes *complete melting* of all particles producing complete cohesion and *maximum volume contraction*. As the liquid is highly viscous, the shape is retained for a short time. If this heating is prolonged the liquid gradually flows under gravity *(pyroplastic flow)* and the article looses sharp corners and shape.

Cooling of the fired article

Firing or heating is discontinued, usually at the high bisque stage after complete melting. Air is allowed to enter the muffle chamber which is gradually cooled, under this air pressure according to the manufacturer's instructions. This is to minimize porosity and the formation of micro-cracks. Then the platform is brought down and the article is cooled and recovered.

Methods to minimize internal porosities

- Firing under vacuum.
- Firing under diffusible gases (H_2 or He having small molecular size).
- Cooling under pressure.

Methods to compensate volume shrinkage

During firing about 30 to 40% volume shrinkage takes place. This is compensated by:

- Applying the slurry (more transparent) on the article and again firing. But repeated firing may reduce the strength.
- Skilled technician prepares about 13% linear oversized condensed pattern (i.e. one-third of 40%) before first firing.

Glazing of fired porcelain articles is *done after applying color frits.*

- To remove the *surface cracks and to improve the flexure strength, glazing is done.*

    Autoglazing or self-glazing: The finished article is kept in the furnace and the temperature is quickly raised (or fired), only to melt the surface particles, which flow and fill all the micro-cracks on the surface which becomes glossy and smooth.

- **Add on or extended glazing:** Special transparent glaze porcelain of *lower fusion temperature* is mixed in water and this slurry is coated on the article as a thin layer. It is then fired at lower temperature to melt only this layer of glaze porcelain, which flows into the surface cracks. Glazing increases the *flexure strength, to nearly double* (from 75 to 135 MPa).

- **Staining:** Color frits of metal oxides are applied to imitate the calcified check-lines before glazing. Color frits and opacifiers to obtain suitable shades, are included in the powder composition.

The entire procedure is complicated and technique sensitive, which demands high skill or training for technicians. Recently simpler CAD-CAM procedure is tried.

10. Explain different types of denture base resin in brief.

Denture is a removable prosthesis that replaces the entire dentition or missing teeth, and associated tissues for normal functions and esthetics. The denture carries the artificial teeth on the base which is supported by thorough contact by the underlying soft tissues. These should satisfy all the requirements such as biocompatibility, physical, mechanical, thermal and esthetics properties. In addition, fabricating technique must be simple and inexpensive. Formerly vulcanite, bakelite, etc., was used. At present polymethyl methacrylate-heat cure, cold cure, or light cure varieties are used with different techniques (compression, injection, fluid resin, etc.). *Note: This introduction required for an essay question).*

Heat cure acrylic-denture base material: Supplied as fine powder or beads of PMMA with benzoyl peroxide initiator, copolymers, dybutyl phthalate as plasticizer, color pigments or fibers. Liquid is methyl methacrylate monomer with co monomers, glycol di-methacrylate as cross-linking agent, and hydroquinone inhibitor to increase shelf-life. These are mixed and packed into the mould (dewaxed space) in the dough stage, bench cured for 30 min, heat-cured at 70°C for 8 hr, bench cooled overnight, recovered and finishing is done.

Properties

Satisfies biological and esthetic requirements and the fabrication method is simple and cheap. Actually the mechanical and thermal properties (low-compressive strength = 75 MPa, tensile strength = 65 MPa, surface hardness = 16–18 KHN, high COTE = 80–120 ppm/°C, low thermal conductivity, etc.) are not satisfactory.

Cold-cure acrylics: Finer powder beads, and liquid also contains the chemical activator dimethylparatolluidine. Since the polymerization begins from the instant of mixing, dough-time is shorter. Curing is done in a pressure-chamber at room temperature for about two hours.

Properties

Satisfies biological and esthetic requirements, but slow *yellowing* may take place due to oxidation of residual amine. Due to lower degree of polymerization, the mechanical properties are poorer by about 10% lower than those of heat cure acrylics. The fabrication method is still simpler and cheaper as heating is not required. This has less internal porosity, better dimensional accuracy and fit.

Hence, cold cure acrylics are used, where strength is not of prime importance, such as for denture-repairs, hard denture liners, orthodontic appliances, etc.

- Pour and cure fluid resin has not become popular.
- VLC, denture fabrication technique is more complicated and does not have better properties.
- Microwave curing denture base technique has slightly better properties.

SHORT ANSWERS   5 × 2 = 10 marks

11. Eame's technique

Eame's technique

This is much simple and commonly adopted silver amalgam condensation technique. Use mercury alloy ratio *1:1 by weight. Excess mercury is not squeezed out.* During condensation also, *expressed mercury from each increment is not removed.*

Precautions

- Large force of condensation 1.6–1.7 kg should be applied
- Condenser tips should be of suitable size or shape
- Homogenous condensation is required
- The mercury rich-portion should not be shifted to the boundaries (which may cause mercuroscopic expansion and ditching).
- Sufficient time should be given, before starting contouring, removing excess, finishing, etc.

12. Elastic limit

Elastic limit is the maximum stress up to which the material can undergo complete elastic recovery. These can be tested by applying different loads (stresses) and finding whether strain vanishes on removal or not. In the actual cases, proportional and elastic limits have nearly same values, as they depend on the permanent slipping of lattices.

However, it is almost impossible to measure exactly these critical limiting values or deviations as they depend on the sensitivity or accuracy (least count) of the measuring instruments. Hence, in practice the measurable yield strength is used. *Yield strength* is the stress required to initiate non-elastic, permanent deformation of say 0.1% or 0.2% strain. Yield strengths of 18-8 stainless steel = 1760 MPa, α-Ti = 438 MPa, β-Ti = 930 MPa, etc.

13. Super-cooled liquids

Many liquids and elements solidify at definite temperatures such as water at 0°C, silver at 960.8°C, gold at 1083°C, copper at 1083°C, titanium at 1668°C, etc., at one atmosphere pressure. During solidification, the dendritic crystals grow around the nuclei of crystallization and the temperature remains constant unlike alloys.

Pure liquids can be very carefully cooled, without disturbing below their normal solidification temperatures. For, example, palladium slightly below 1552°C. This is a very **unstable super-cooled state** in which stable nuclei of crystallizations are formed. Greater supercooling, more are the numbers of such nuclei of crystallization, which produce more grains per unit volume, i.e. finer grains resulting in higher strength. This is homogenous nucleation. However, alloys have range of melting temperatures and solidify by **constitutional supercooling** which results in cored structure.

14. Spherulites

When gypsum products are mixed with water the $CaSO_4$ hemihydrate of greater solubility (0.9%), form $CaSO_4$ dihydrate of lower solubility (0.2%) and the solution gets *supersaturated.* These precipitate around the nuclei of uncalcined gypsum impurities, radially and form spherical structures which are called as spherulites. These intermesh with each other producing a rigid mass. The lateral thrust causes setting expansions. The strength of set material and the setting expansions are more if the number of spherulites per unit volume (i.e. nuclei of crystallization) is more (i.e. lower W/P ratio). The reaction rate increases and setting time decreases. The manufacturer and technicians can easily control these aspects.

15. Die spacers

During lost-wax casting procedures, all precautions and methods are applied to compensate casting shrinkages very accurately. Due to this, there may not be any space left out, for cementation. To retain a thin cementation space, die spacers used.

One or a few thin coatings (7–10 microns) of nail paints, resin paints or some cellulose suspensions of gold or silver colors (Trade name *Pico-fit*) are used. Sometimes die enlargement technique is also used.

Colour plates with references for practical-spotters and dental materials practicals

Part I

Plate 1

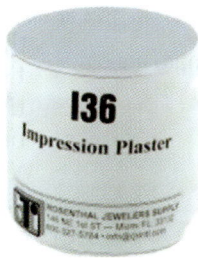

Fig. 1: Impression plaster

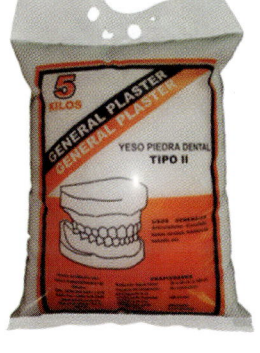

Fig. 2: Model plaster

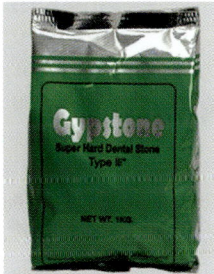

Fig. 3: Dental stone

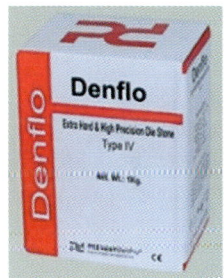

Fig. 4: Type IV die stone

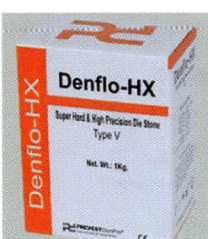
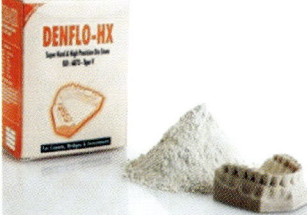

Fig. 5: Type V die stone

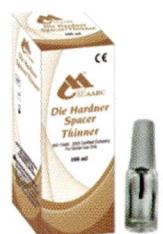

Fig. 5a: Die spacer

Plate 2

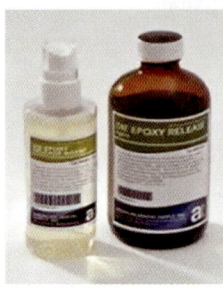

Fig. 5b: Epoxy resin die material

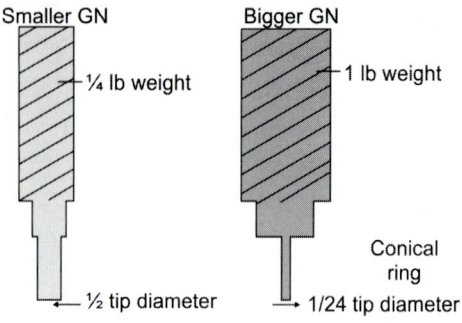

Fig. 6: Gilmore needle

Smaller GN

¼ lb weight

½ tip diameter

Bigger GN

1 lb weight

Conical ring

1/24 tip diameter

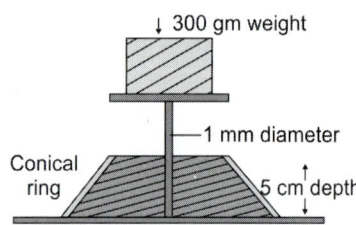

↓ 300 gm weight

1 mm diameter

Conical ring

5 cm depth

Fig. 7: Vicat penetrometer

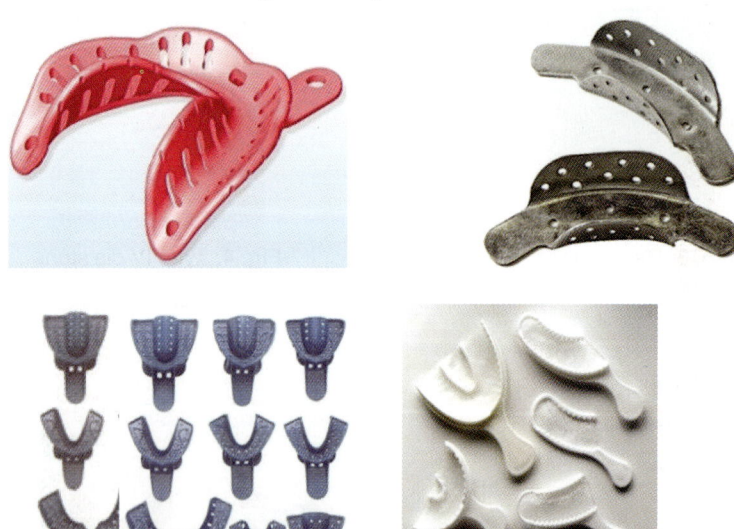

Plate 3

(Contd.)

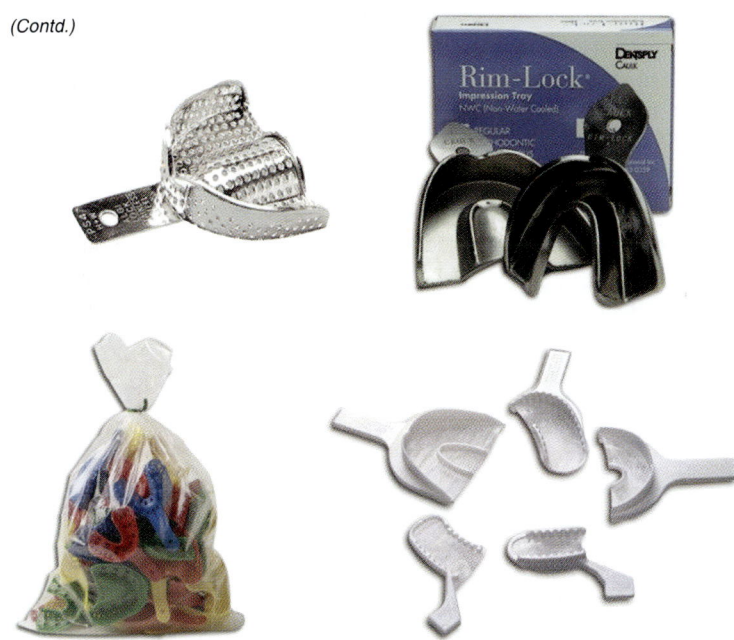

Fig. 8: Impression trays (varieties)

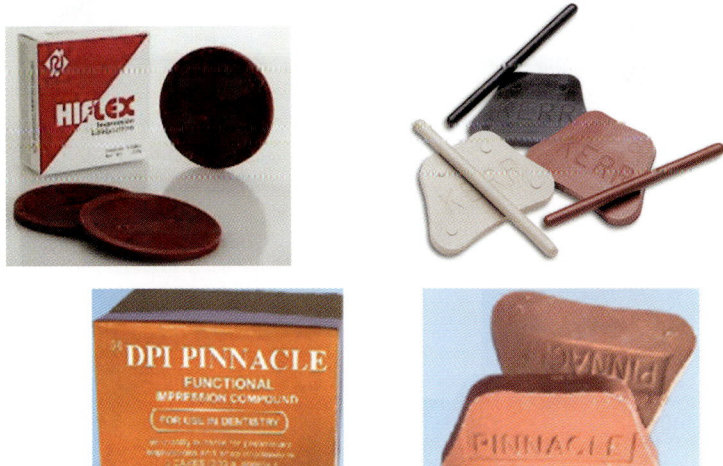

Fig. 9: Type I: Low fusing impression compound

Plate 4

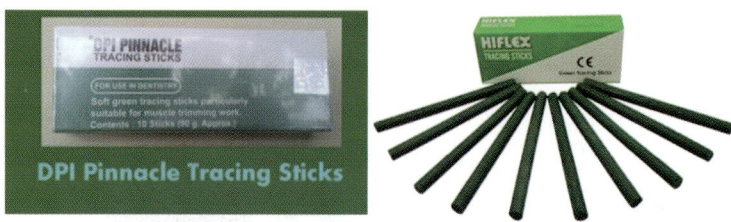

Fig. 10: Type I: Greenstick compound (tracing compound)

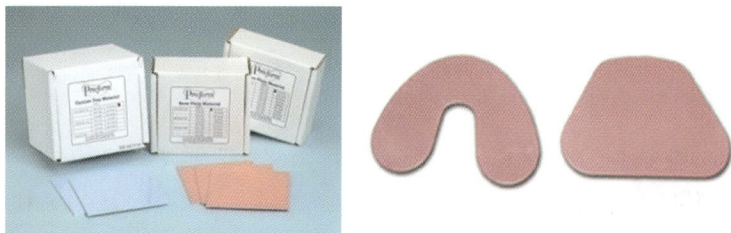

Fig. 10a: Shellac base plate

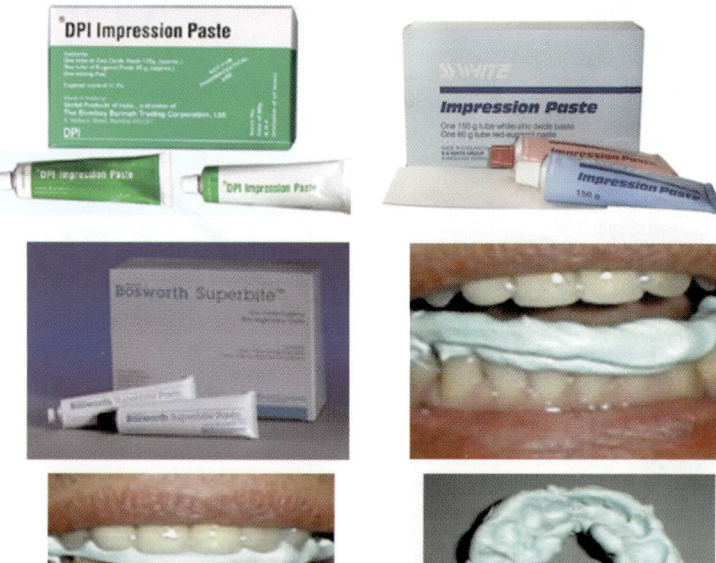

Fig. 11: Zinc oxide eugenol impression paste, bite registration paste (functional impression) as shown in the diagram

Plate 5

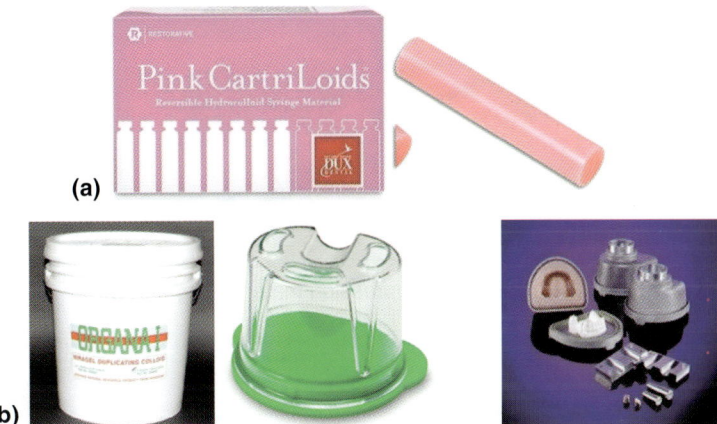

Fig. 12: (a) Agar-agar impression material supplied in syringe form, (b) supplied tin or Jar for duplicating procedures along with duplicating flask

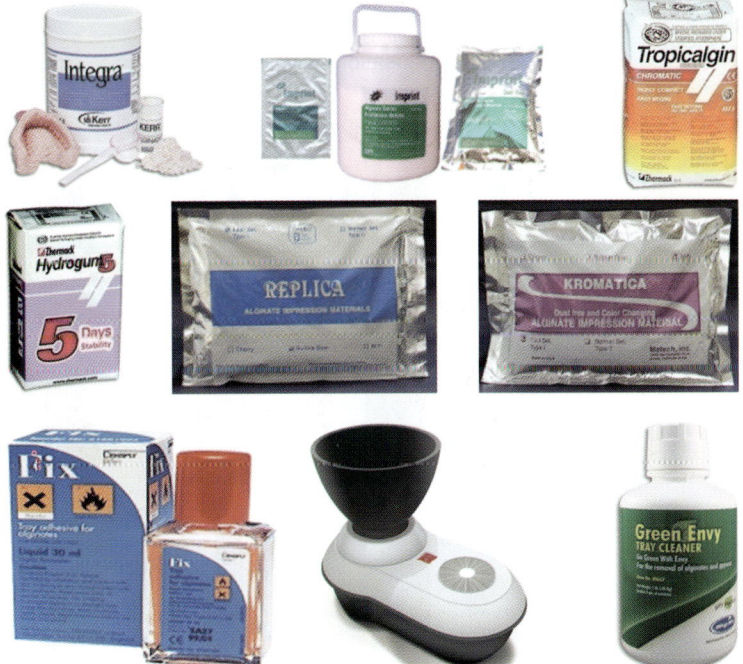

Fig. 13: Various brands of alginate impression material along with tray adhesive and mechanical mixing device

Plate 6

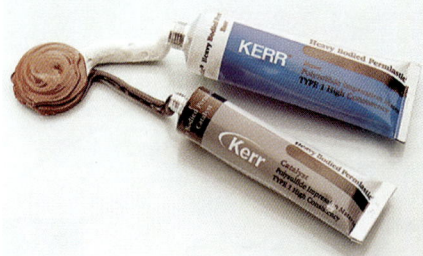

Fig. 14: Polysulphide impression material—light body

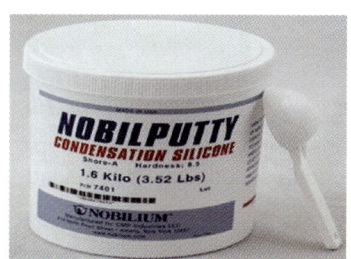 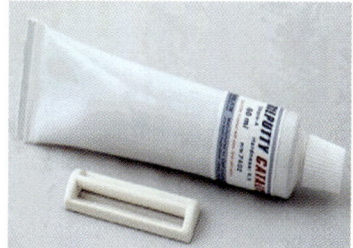

Fig. 15: Condensation polysilicone

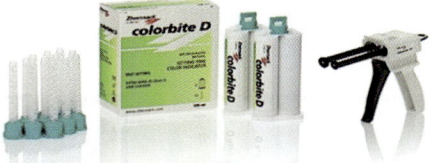

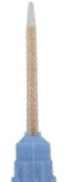 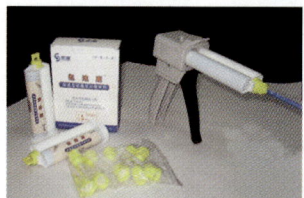 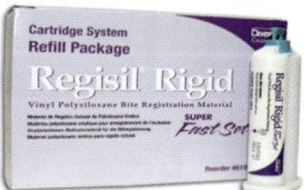

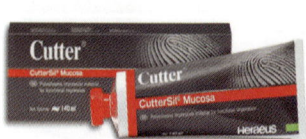 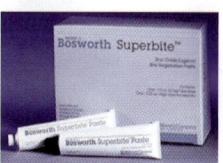 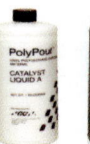 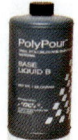

Fig. 16: Addition polysilicone supplied in cartridge system and also two-paste system, for bite registration, and duplicating

Plate 7

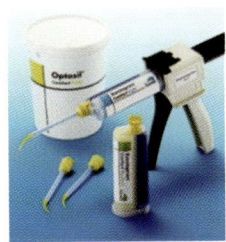

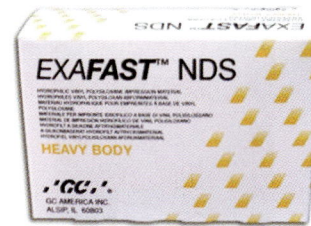

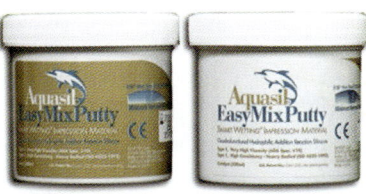

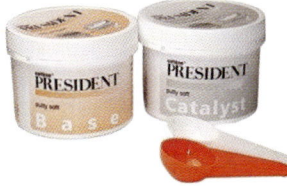

Fig. 16a: Addition polysilicone impression material—putty consistency, light body supplied in cartridge for automixing (left top)

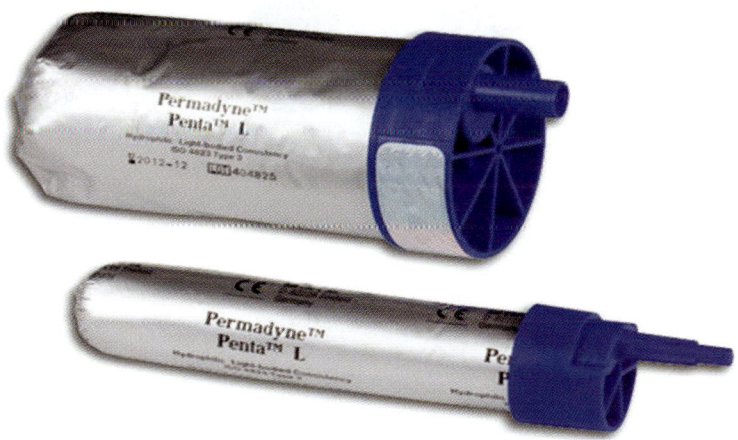

Fig. 17: Polyether impression material—light activated

Plate 8

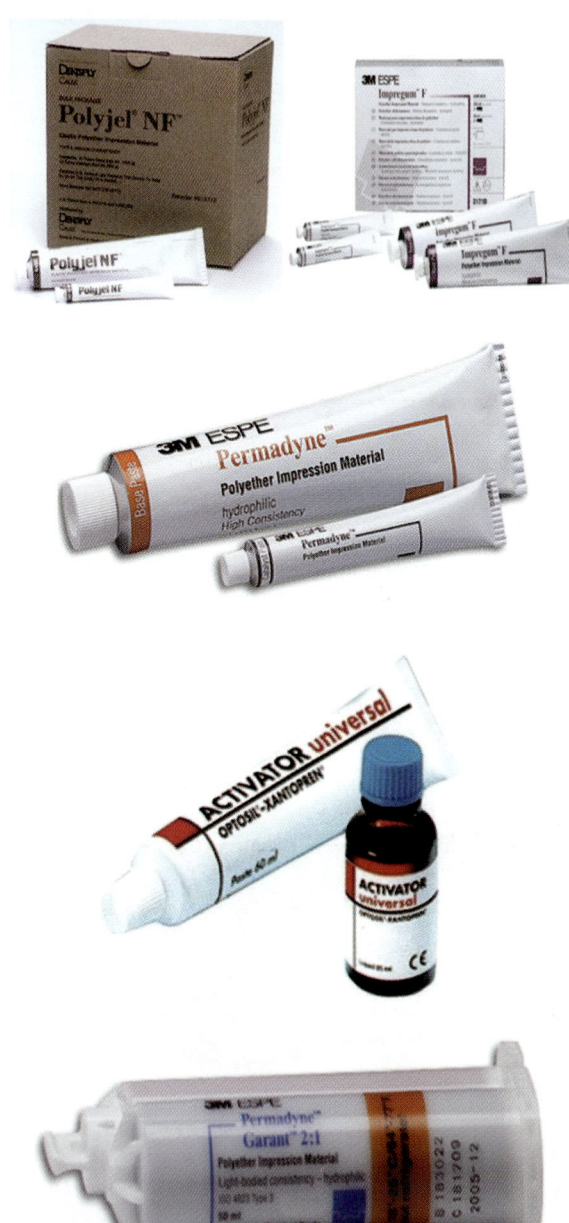

Fig. 17b: Polyether impression material—chemical activated

Plate 9

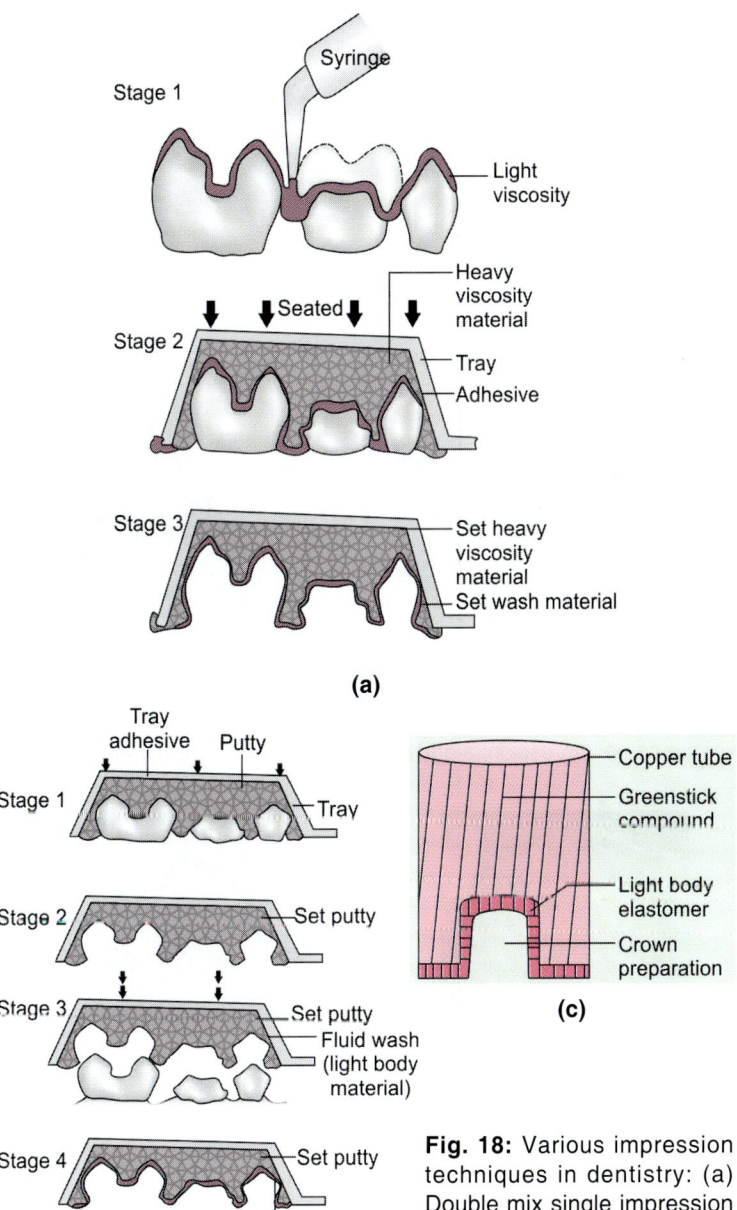

Fig. 18: Various impression techniques in dentistry: (a) Double mix single impression technique, (b) double mix-double mix (relive), (c) copper tube impression

Plate 10

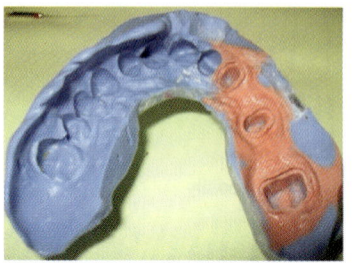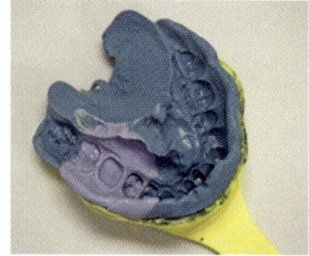

Fig. 18a: Double mix single impression technique by using medium or heavy body with light body

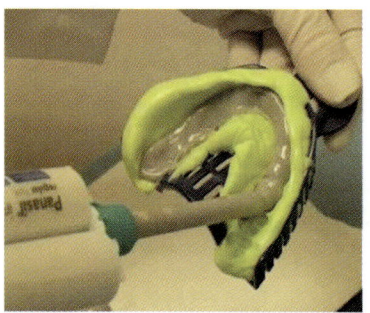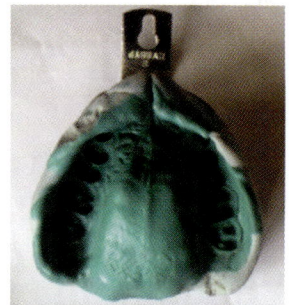

Fig. 18b: Double mix double impression by using putty body in stock trays recording primary impression and later recording secondary with light body over the same impression; a and b prepared from different brands

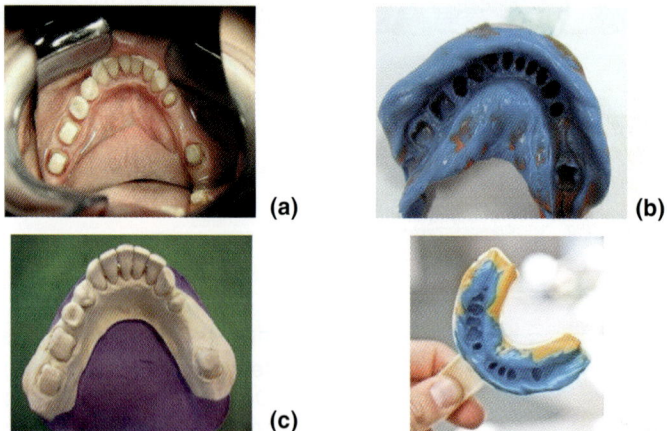

(a)

(b)

(c)

Fig. 18c: (a) Patient oral cavity—prepared tooth, (b) impression (single mix single impression technique), (c) cast

Plate 11

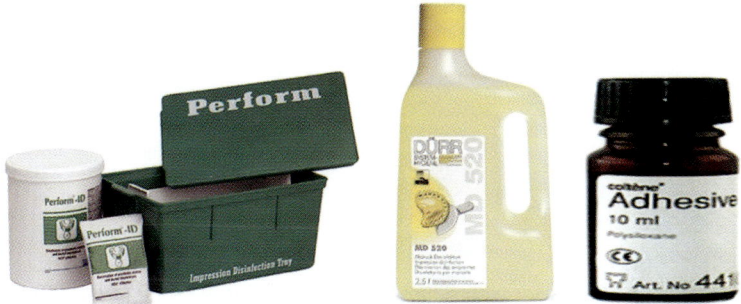

Fig. 18d: Impression disinfectant solution, tray adhesive for elastomer

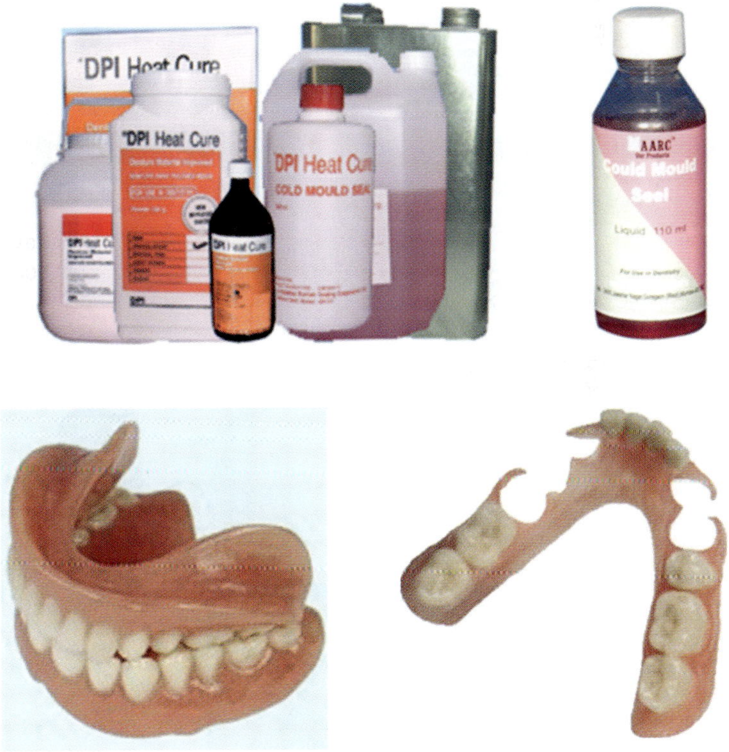

Fig. 19: Polymethyl methacrylate denture base material supplied as powder and liquid (in amber-colored bottle or tin, separating medium (pink color), used for complete denture and partial denture fabrication

Plate 12

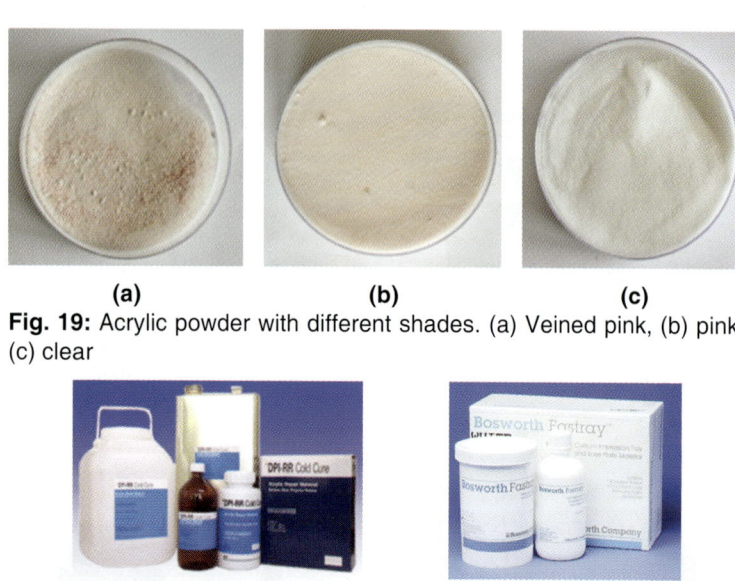

(a) **(b)** **(c)**

Fig. 19: Acrylic powder with different shades. (a) Veined pink, (b) pink, (c) clear

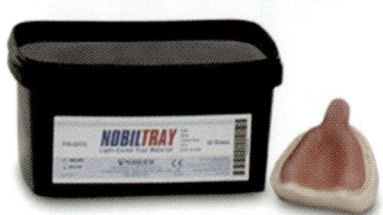
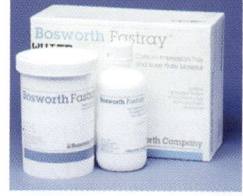
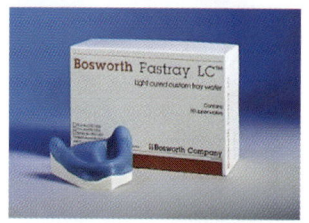
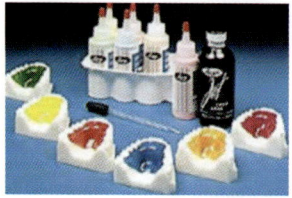
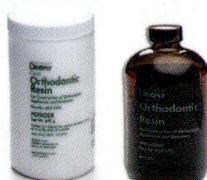
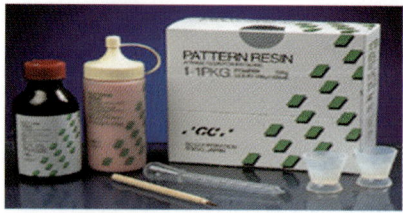

Fig. 20: Self cure acrylic resin, light cure for tray fabrication, orthodontic appliances, pattern preparation for investing

Plate 13

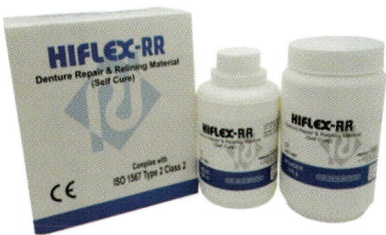

Fig. 21: Repair resins

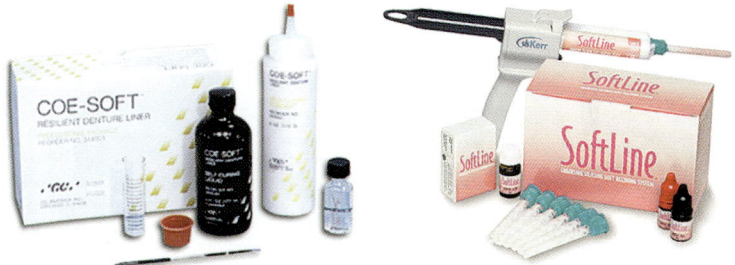

Fig. 22: Soft denture liners

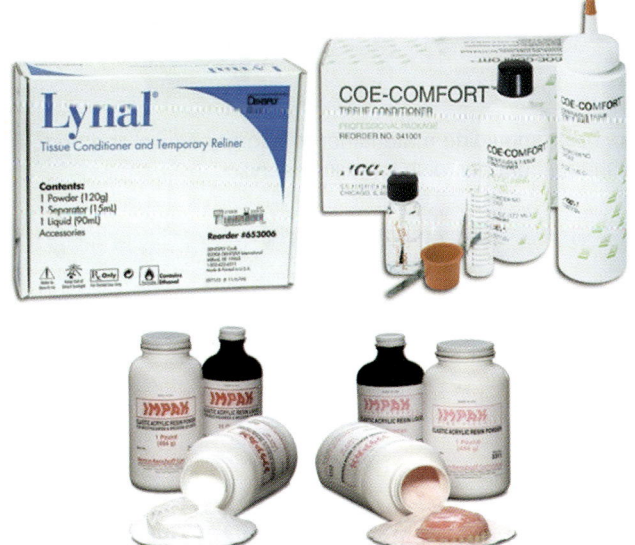

Fig. 23: Tissue conditioner with different shades

Plate 14

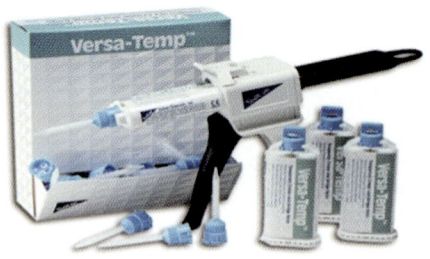
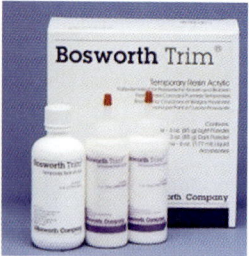

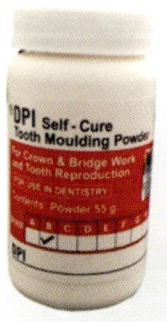
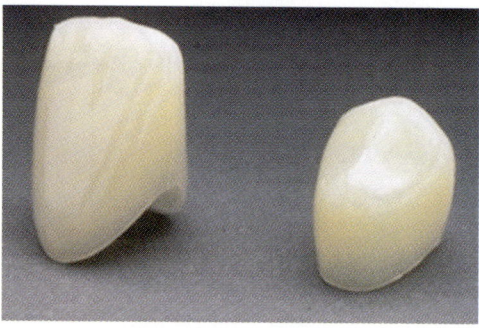

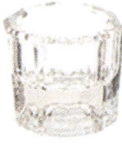
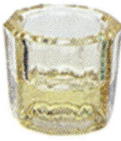
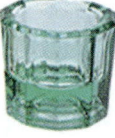

Fig. 24a: Tooth moulding material for temporary crown and bridge with different shades, dappen dish for mixing acrylic

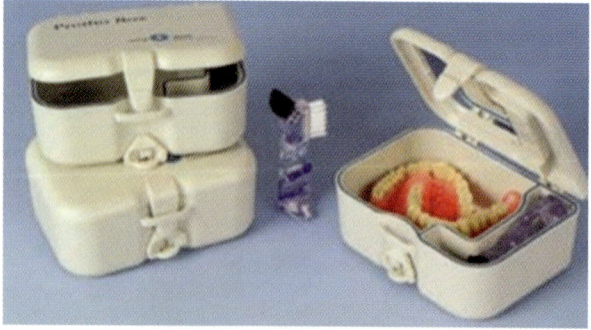

Fig. 24b: Denture kit for patient

Plate 15

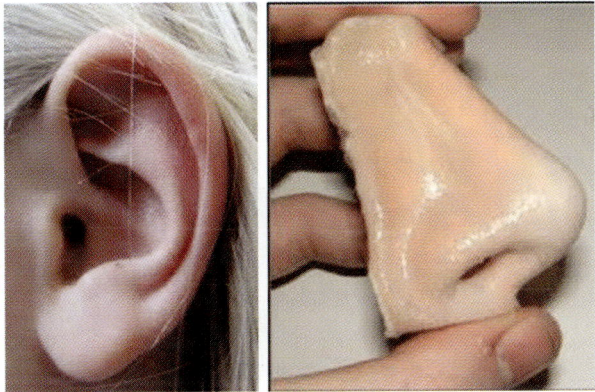

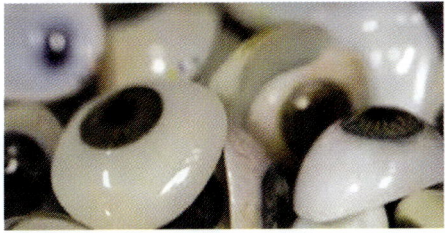

Fig. 25: Maxillofacial appliances: Ear, nose, eye shell

Part II

Plate 16

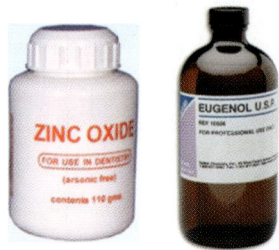

Fig. 26: Conventional ZnOE dental cement

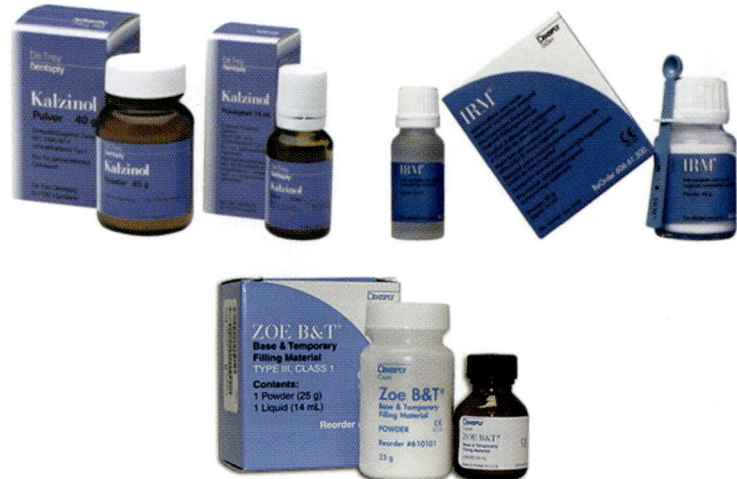

Fig. 27a: Resin modified ZnOE cement (brands—Kalzinol and IRM)

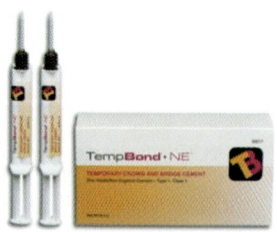

Fig. 27b: Type I ZnOE—dispensed in cartridge for easy mixing

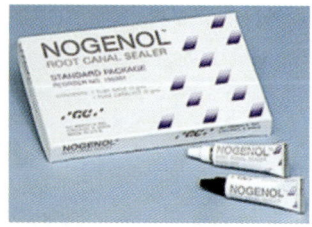

Fig. 28: Non-eugenol cement (alumima based—EBA)

Plate 17

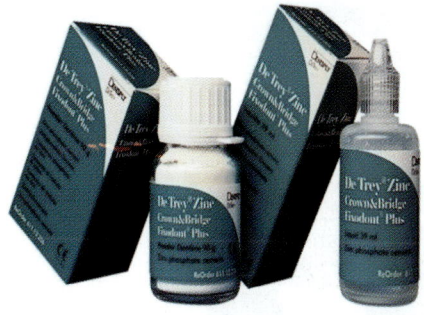
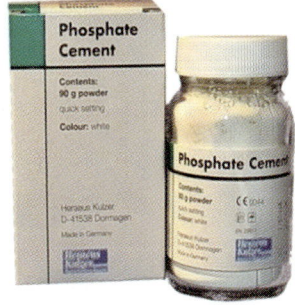

Fig. 29: Zinc phosphate cement (brand—De Trey)

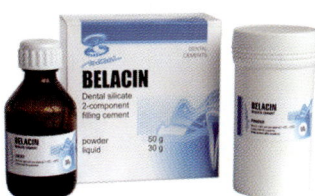
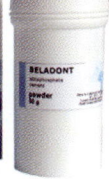

Fig. 30: Silicate cement   **Fig. 31:** Zinc silicophosphate cement

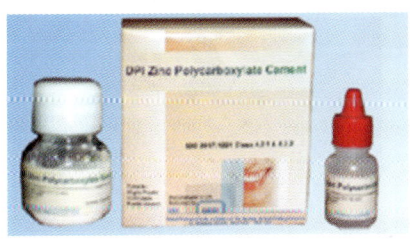
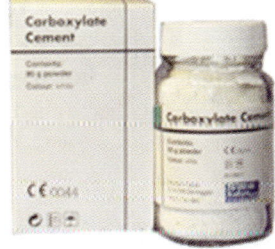

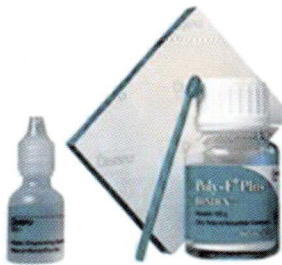
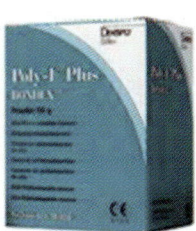

Fig. 32: Zinc polycarboxylate cement (brand—Poly F)

Plate 18

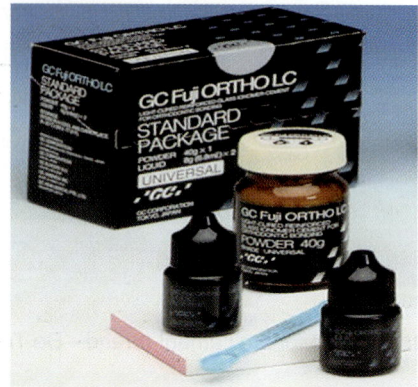

Fig. 33: Glass ionomer cement type I—cementation material

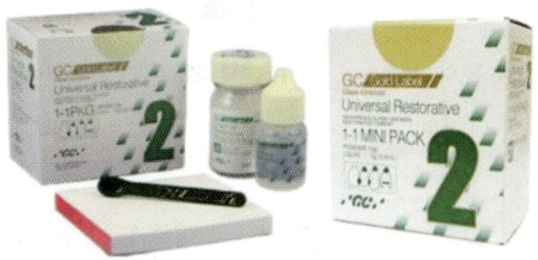

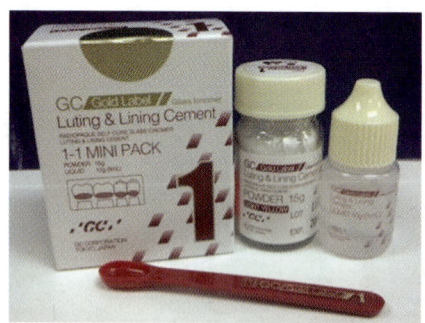
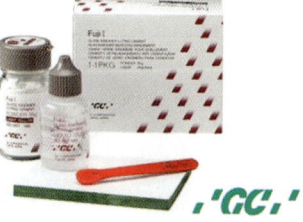

Fig. 34: Glass ionomer cement type II—restorative material

Plate 19

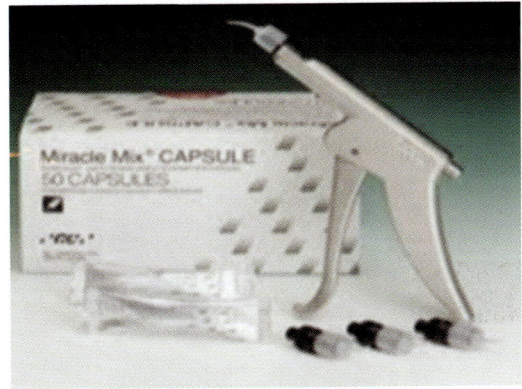

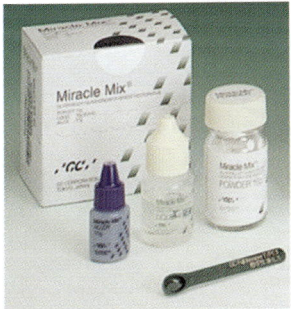

Fig. 35: Metal modified GIC (brand—Miracle mix)

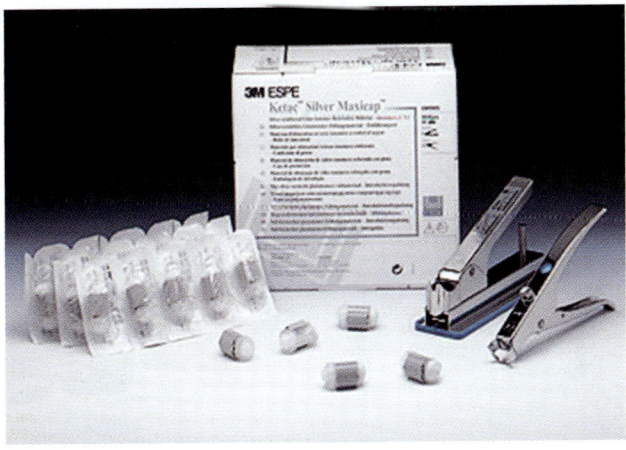

Fig. 36: Metal modified GIC (brand—Ketac Siver)

Plate 20

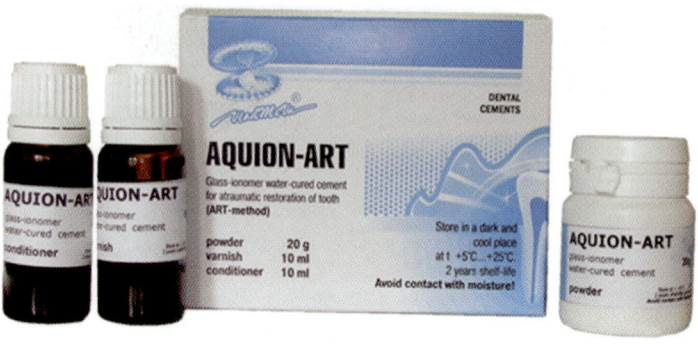

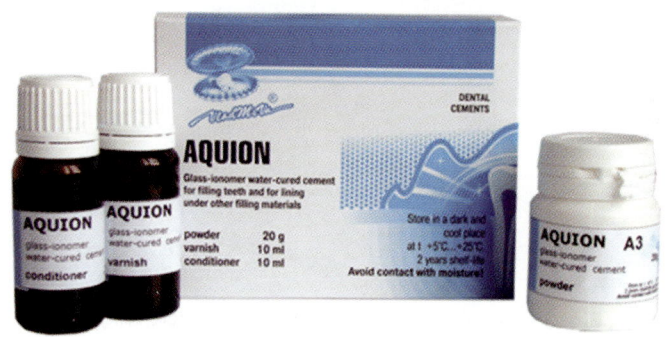

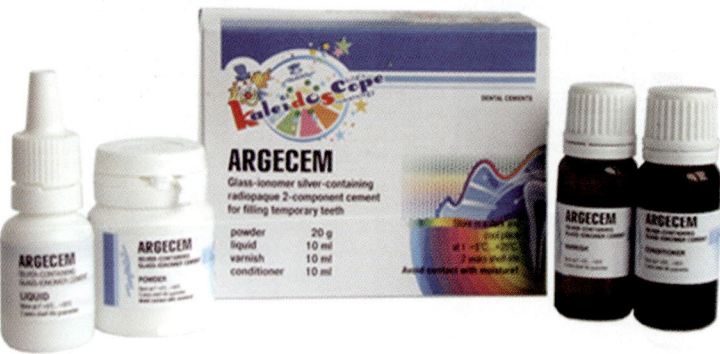

Fig. 36a: "Argecem" (Ag) metal modified cermet

Plate 21

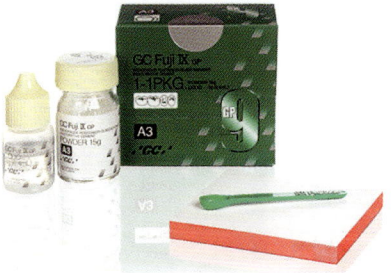

Fig. 37: GIC type IX restorative material (for pediatric and gediatric)

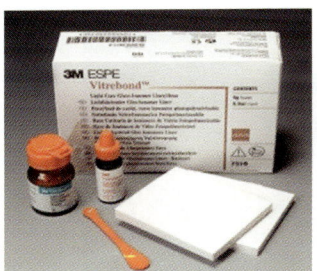

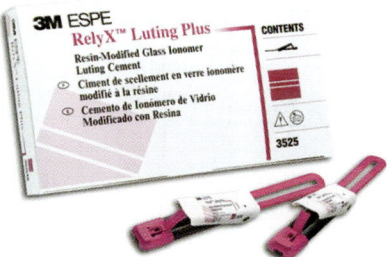

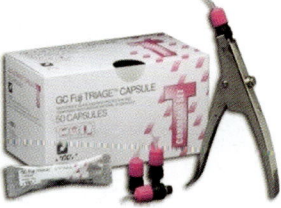

Fig. 38: Resin modified glass ionomer cement

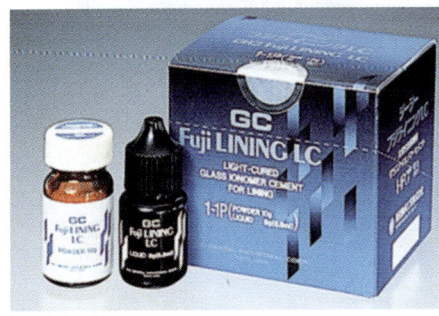

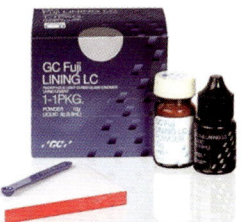

Fig. 38(a): Type III—Light curable GIC liner

Plate 22

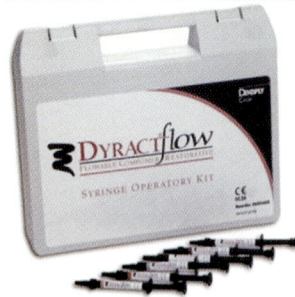 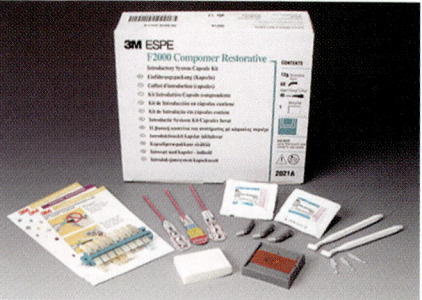

Fig. 39: Compomer restorative material

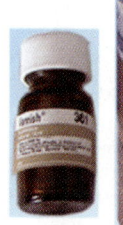 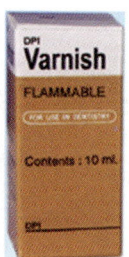 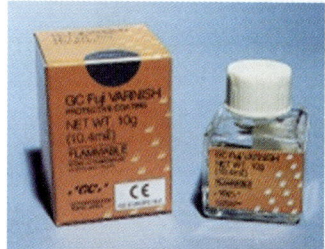

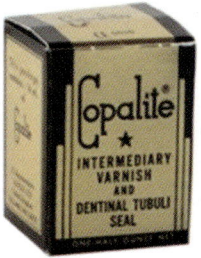 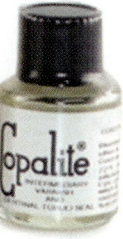 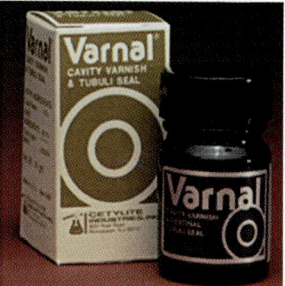

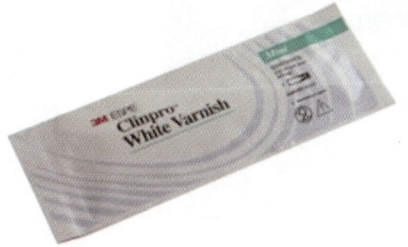

Fig. 40: Cavity varnish

Plate 23

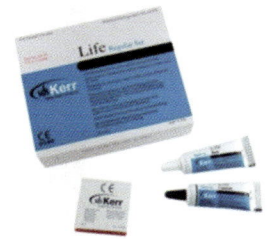

Fig. 41: Cavity liner or pulp capping agent $(Ca(OH)_2)$

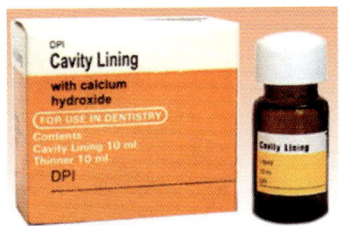

Fig. 42: Cavity liner

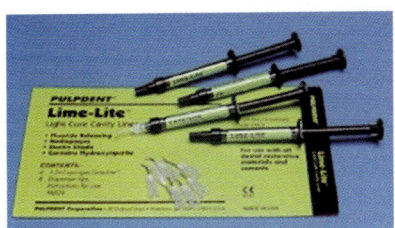

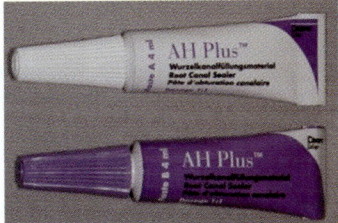

Fig. 42a: Calcium hydroxide cement

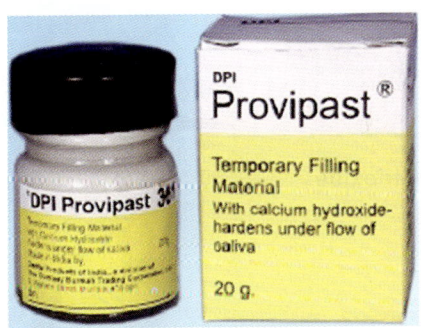

Fig. 42b: Single paste system in $Ca(OH)_2$

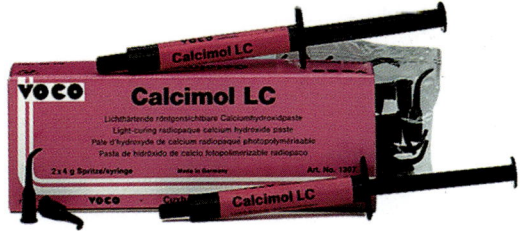

Fig. 42c: Light curable calcium hydroxide cement

Plate 24

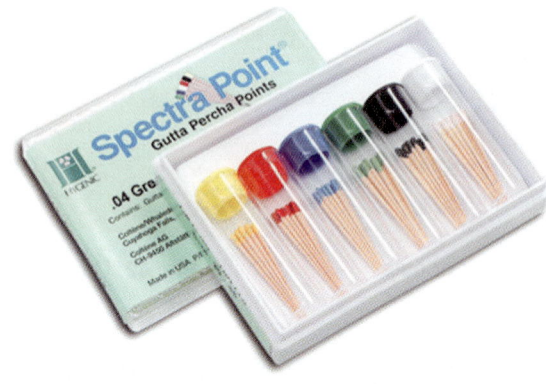

Fig. 43: Gutta-percha points

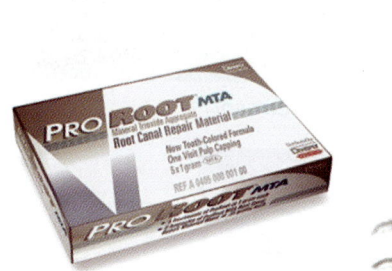

Fig. 44: Mineral trioxide (MTA)

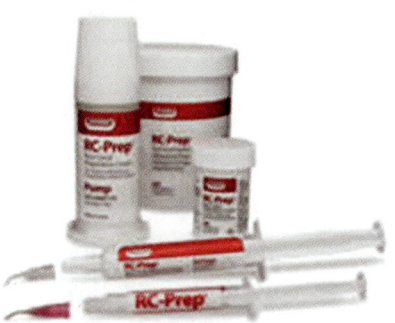

Fig. 45: RC prep

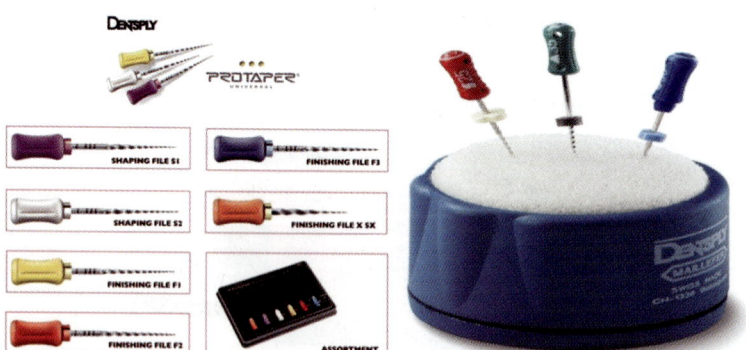

Fig. 45a: Endodontic files

Plate 25

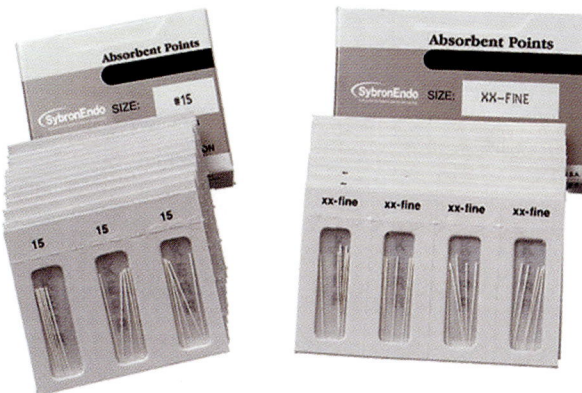

Fig. 45b: Paper points

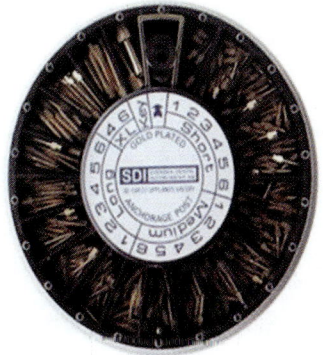

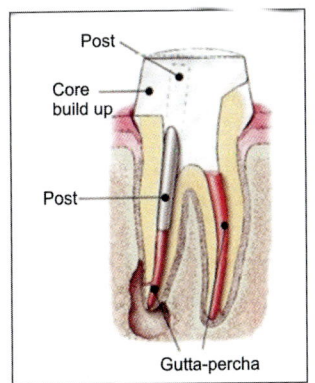

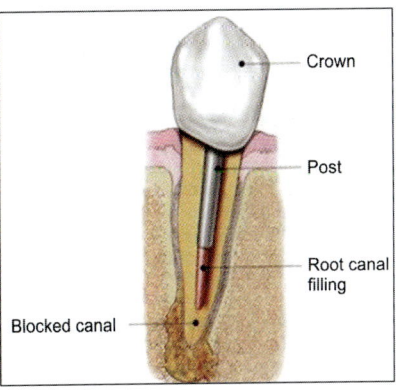

Fig. 45c: Preformed post and core of various sizes

Plate 26

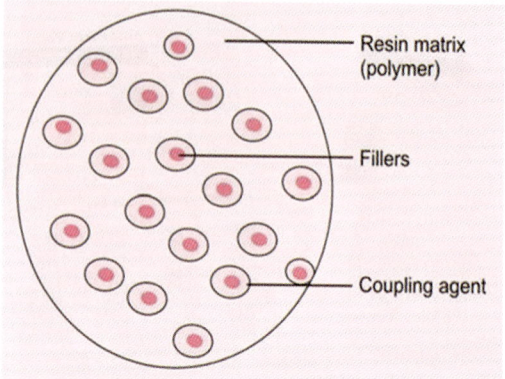

Fig. 46: Structure of composite resins

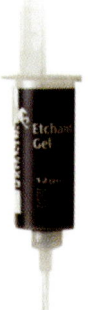
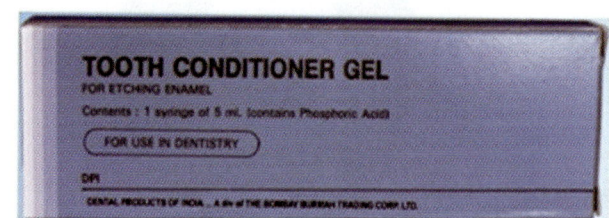

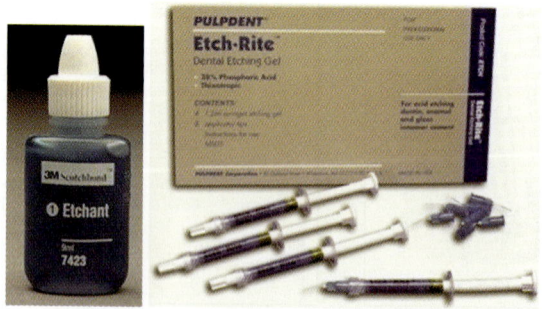

Fig. 47: Acid etchants for compsite resin

Plate 27

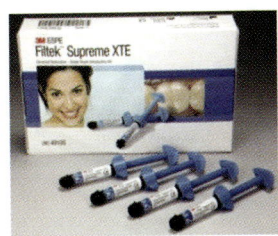 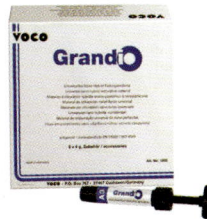 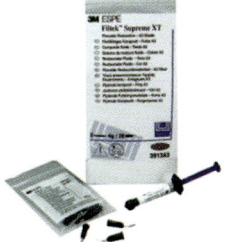

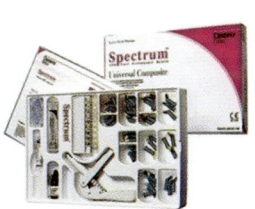 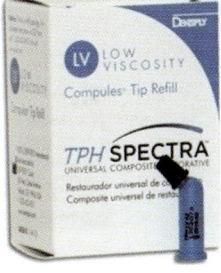 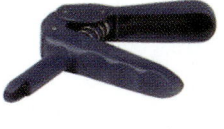

Fig. 48: Composite resin varieties—light cure also supplied with discharge gun for capsule system

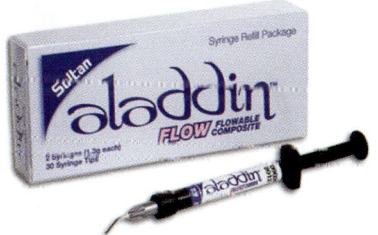 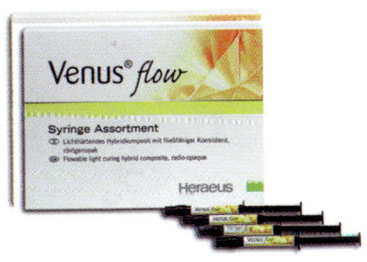

Fig. 48a: Flowable composite

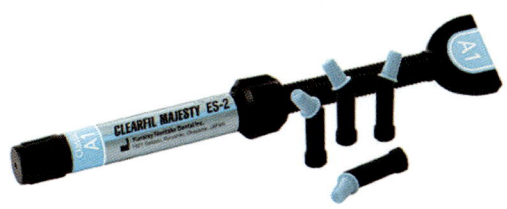

Fig. 48b: Nanocomposite

Plate 28

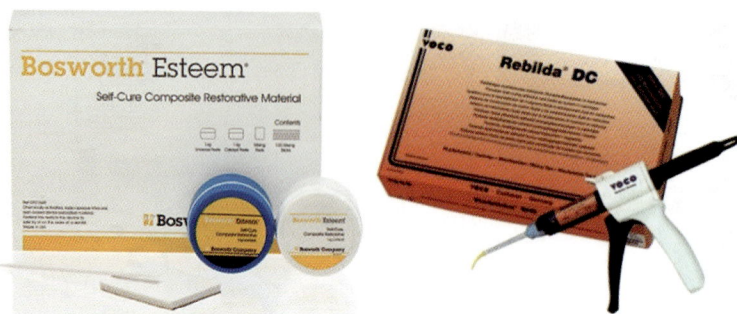

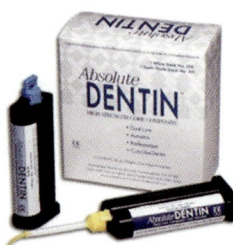

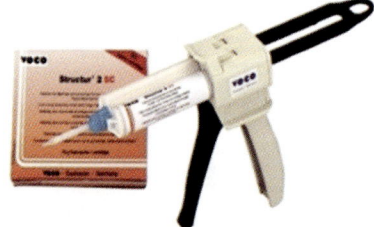

Fig. 48c: Composite resin varieties—self cure

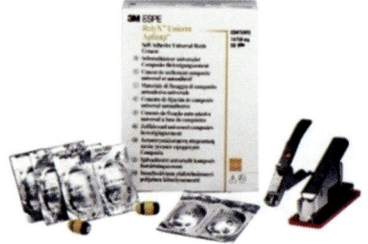

Fig. 48d: Self adhesive universal resin cement

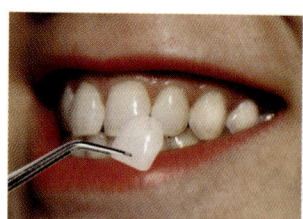

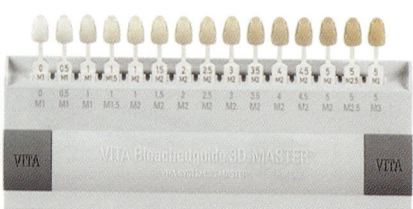

Fig. 48e: Shade guide

Plate 29

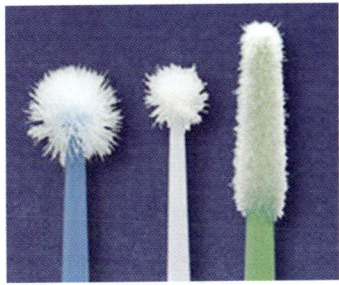

Fig. 48f: Applicator tip (brush) for bonding agents

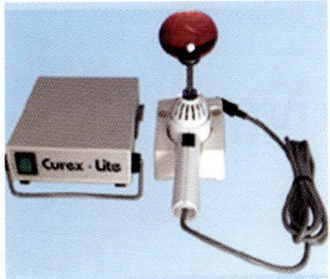

Fig. 48g: Light curing unit for composite resins

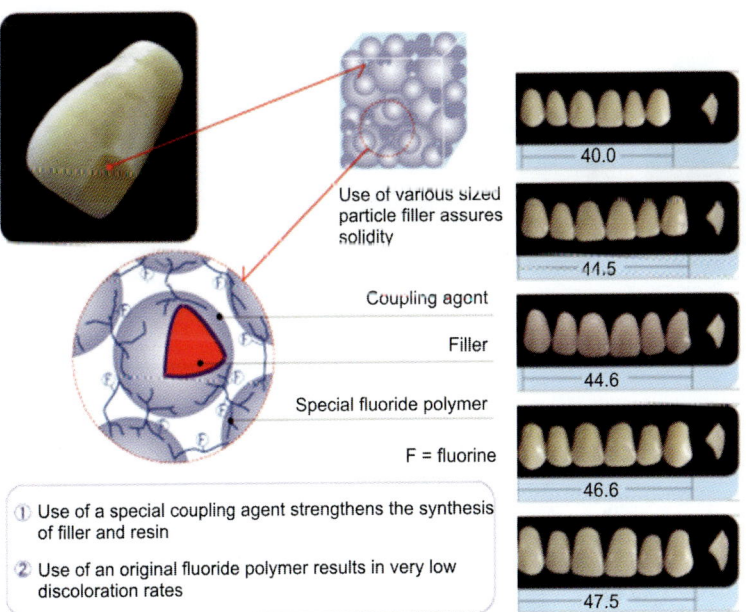

Fig. 48h: Bonding agents varieties

Plate 30

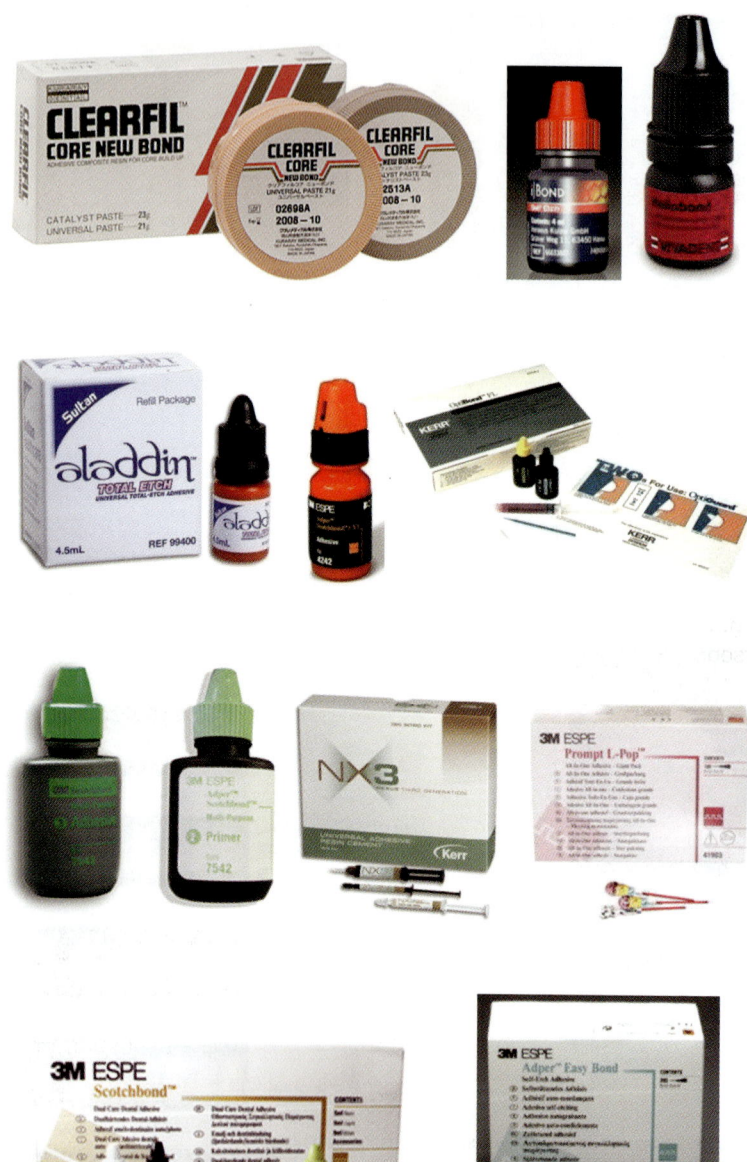

Fig. 48i: Bonding agents varieties

Plate 31

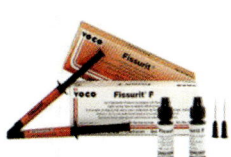 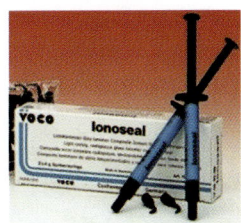 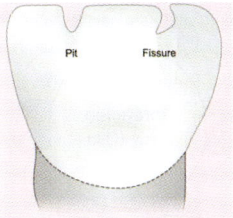

Fig. 49: Pit and fissure sealants

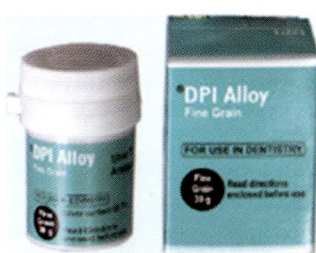 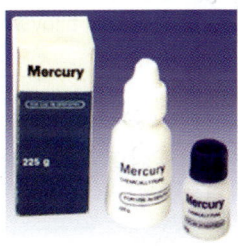

Fig. 50: Low copper silver amalgam alloy powder and triple distilled arsenic-free mercury

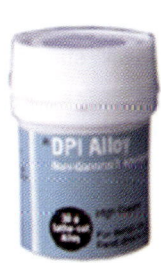 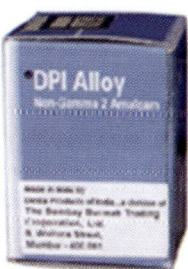 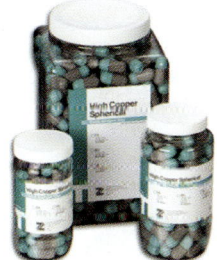

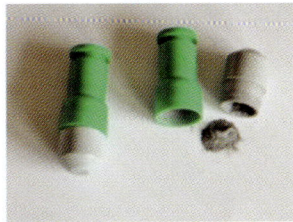

Fig. 51: High copper silver amalgam alloy powder (non-gamma 2) and triple distilled arsenic-free mercury, also available in capsule form

Plate 32

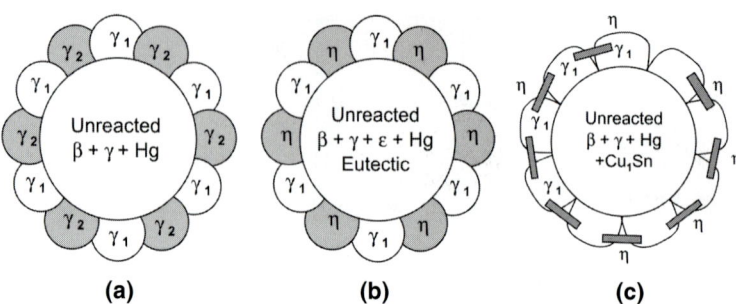

(a)   **(b)**   **(c)**

Fig. 52a to c : Microstructure of low copper, high copper, admixed and single composition alloys

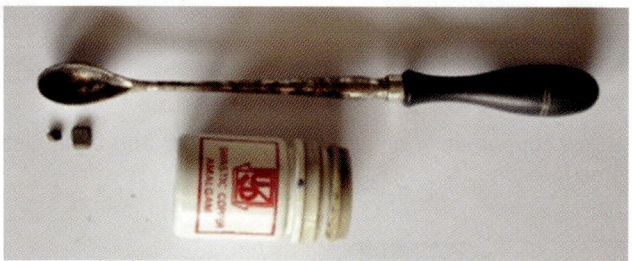

Fig. 53: Copper amalgam supplied in pellate form along with stainless steel spatula for manipulation

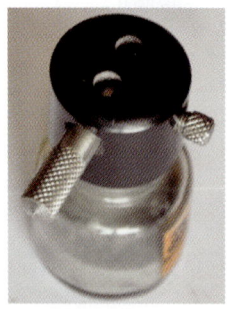

Fig. 54a: Amalgam alloy dispenser

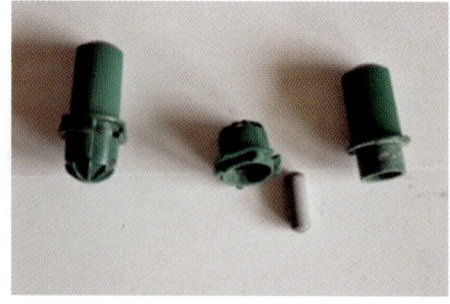

Fig. 54b: Pestle in capsule, for mechanical mixing

Plate 33

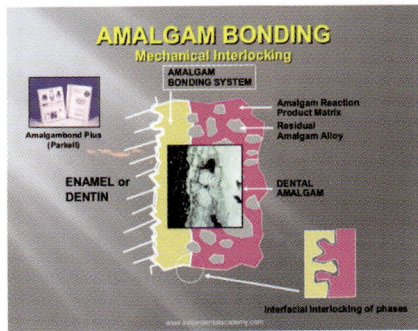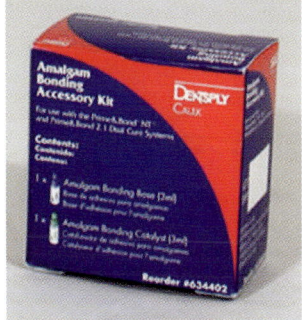

Fig. 55: Amalgam bond

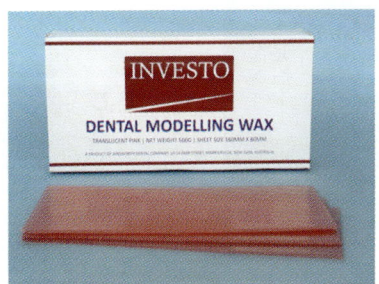

Fig. 56: Modelling wax

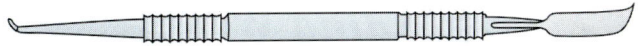

Fig. 56a: Wax carver

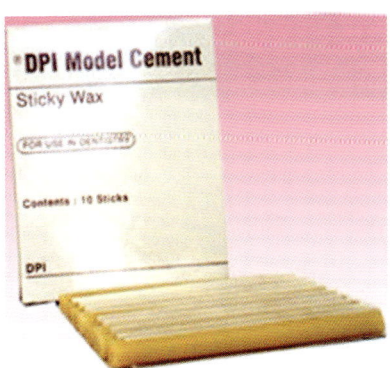

Fig. 57: Sticky wax

Plate 34

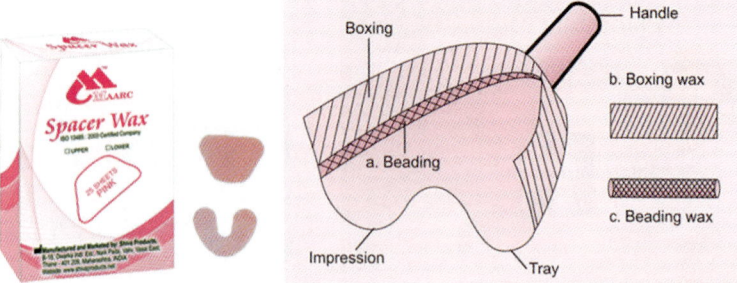

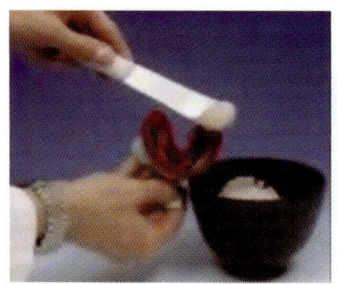

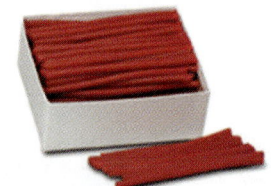

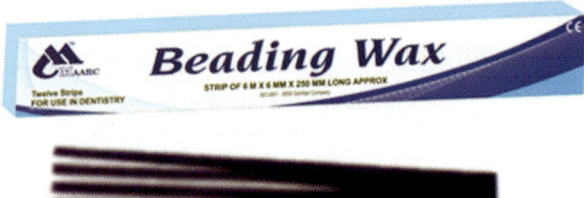

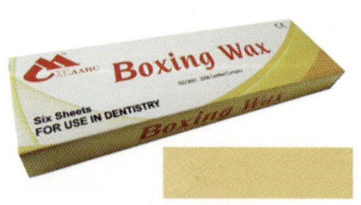

Fig. 58: Beading wax and boxing wax

Plate 35

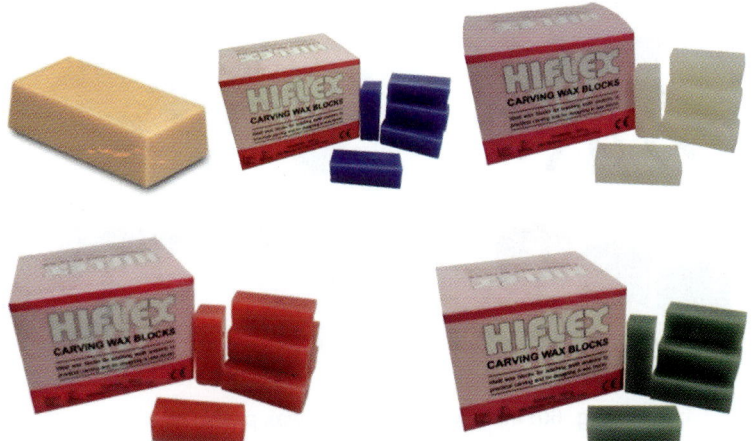

Fig. 59: Carving wax with different colors

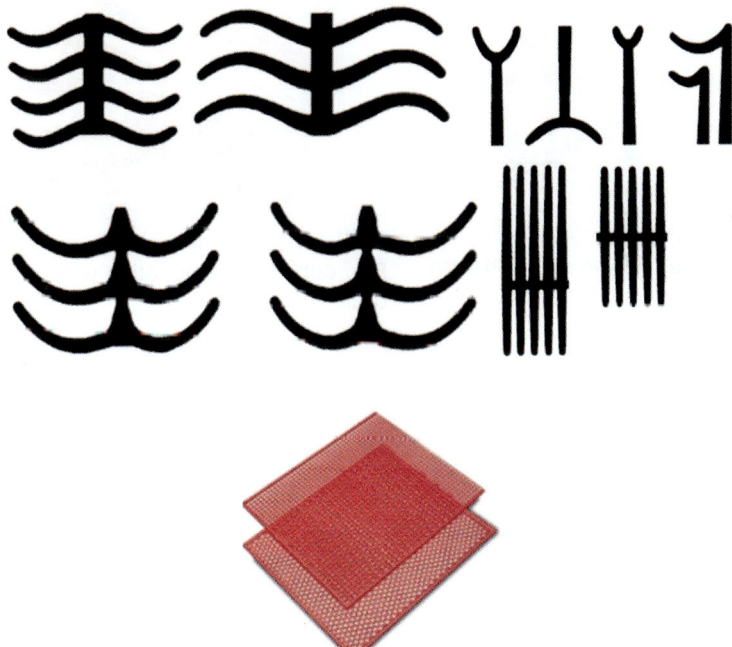

Fig. 59a: Casting wax to fabricate metal framework for cast partial denture

Plate 36

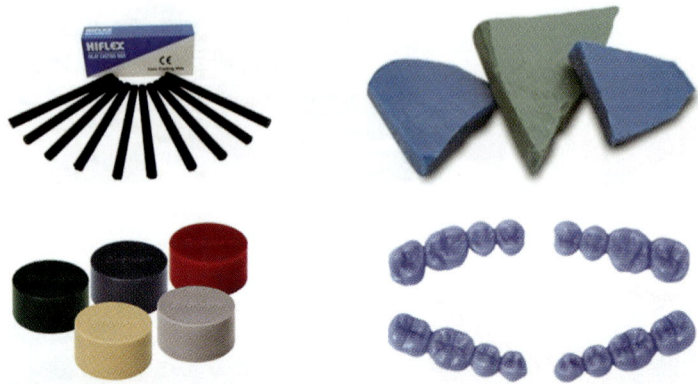

Fig. 60: Inlay wax, preformed wax patterns

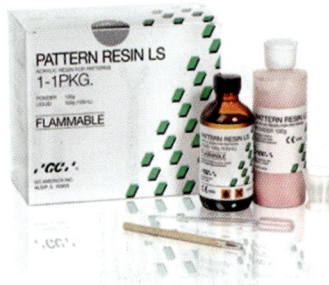

Fig. 60a: Acrylic resin (PMMA) for pattern fabrication

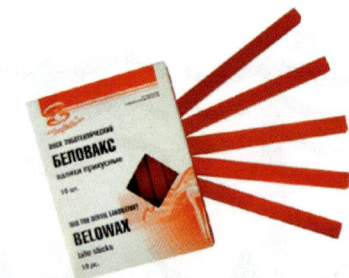

Fig. 60b: Bite registration wax for occlusal relations

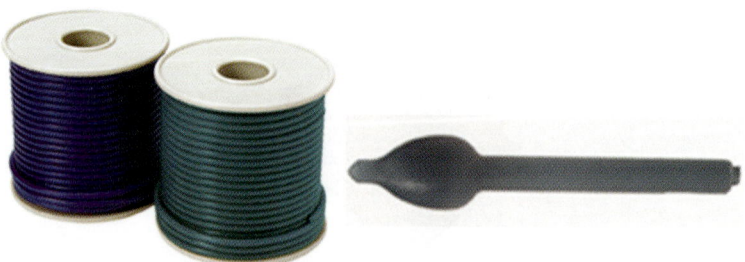

Fig. 61: Sprue former

Plate 37

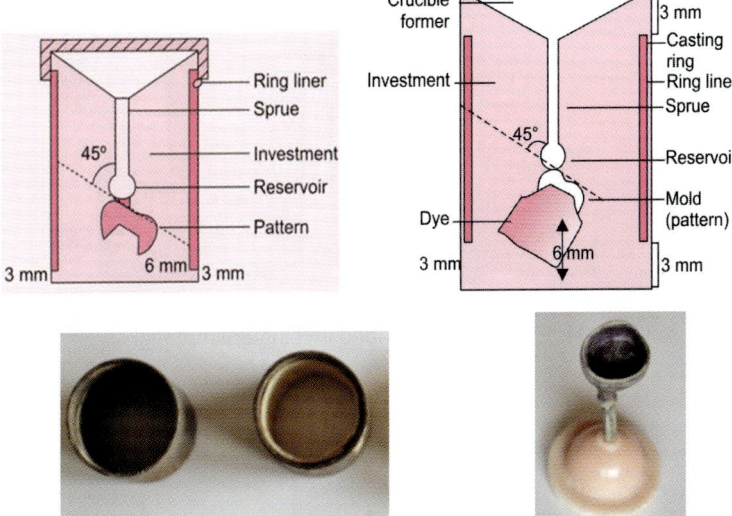

Fig. 62: Cross section of (a) invested and (b) divested casting ring, (c) ring liner, (d) direct sprued wax pattern with crucible former

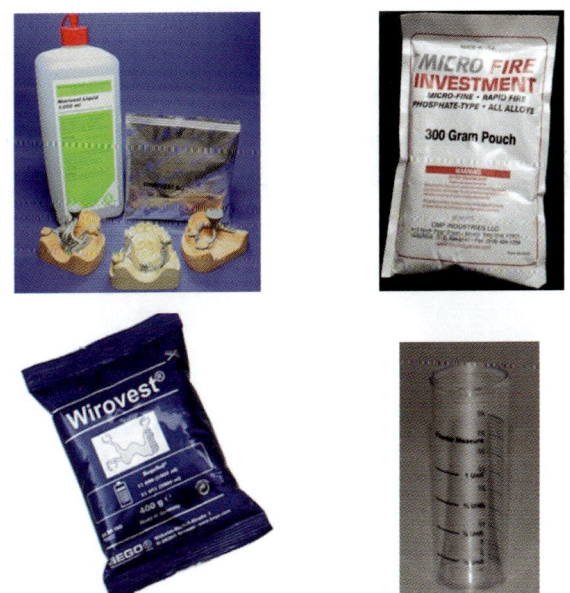

Fig. 63: Phosphate bonded investment material

Plate 38

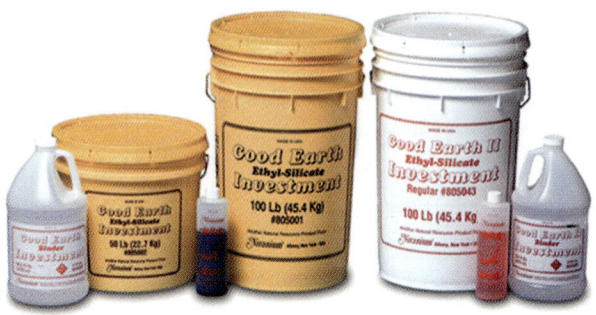

Fig. 64: Ethyl silicate bonded investment material

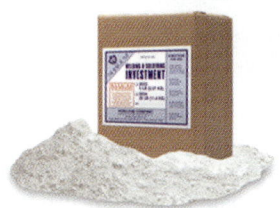

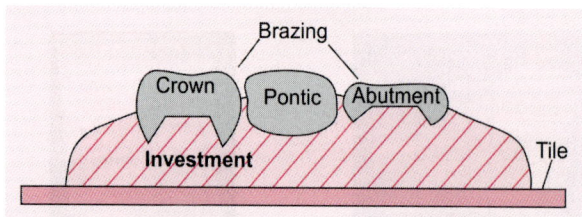

Fig. 65: Soldering investment material

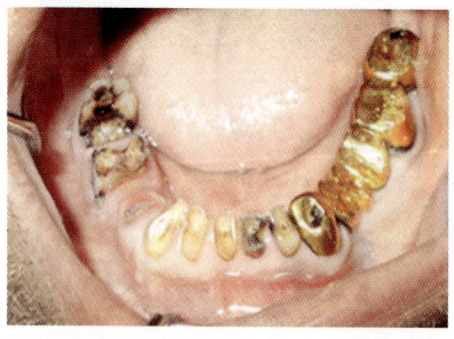

Fig. 66: Japanese gold or technique alloy (yellow metal)

Plate 39

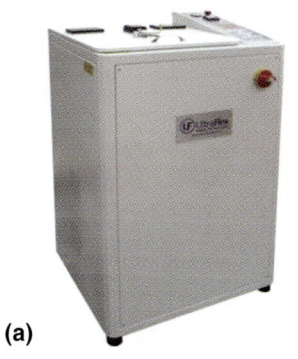

(a)

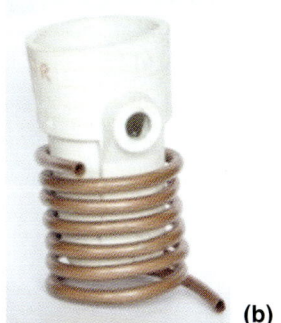

(b)

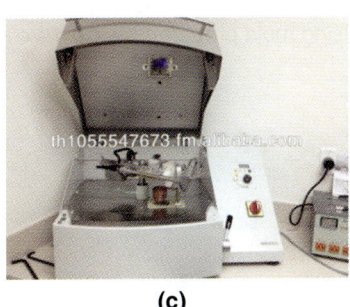

(c)

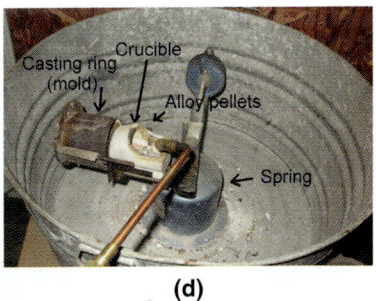

(d)

Fig. 67: (a) Induction casting machine, (b) crucible placed in induction coil, (c) inner views of induction and (d) gas melting casting machine

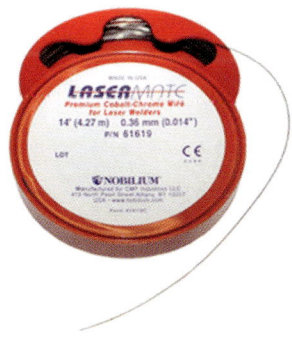

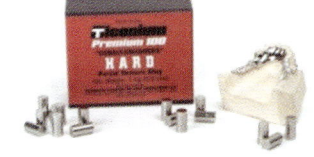

Fig. 68a: Co-Cr orthodontic wire   **Fig. 68b:** PBM casting alloy pellets

Plate 40

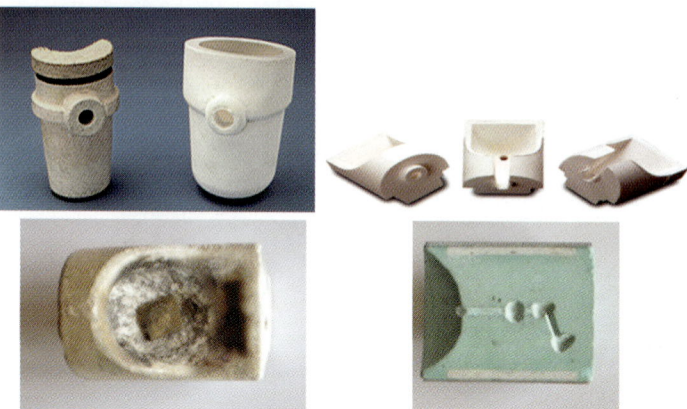

Fig. 69: Casting crucible for induction casting and gas torch melting (pellet is placed in the crucible and casted by using mold prepared by lost wax casting procedure)

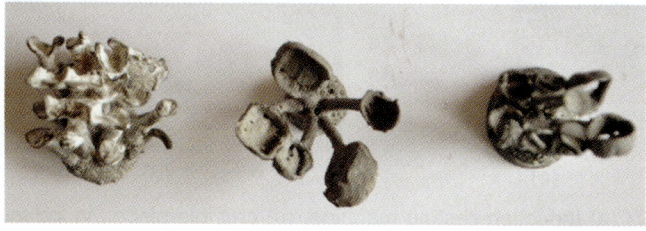

Fig. 70: Casting defects: Incomplete casting, surface roughness, etc.

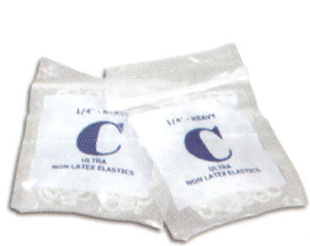

Fig. 71a: Orthodontic bands

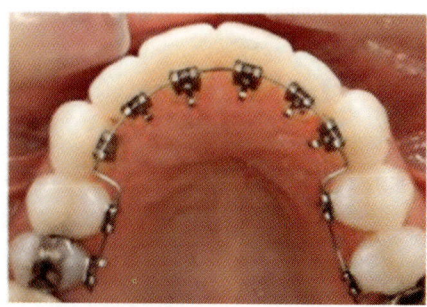

Fig. 71b: Orthodontic lingual side appliances

Plate 41

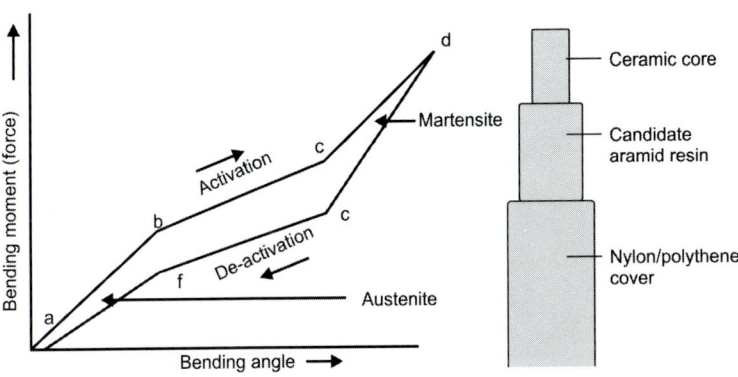

Fig. 72: Ni-Ti orthodontic wire (phase changes) superelasticity

Fig. 73: Aesthetic orthodontic wire

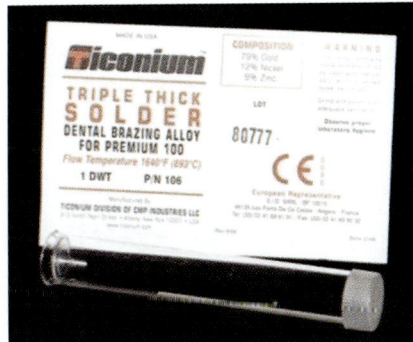

Fig. 74: Solder (Comp 79% Au, 12% Ni and 9% Zn)

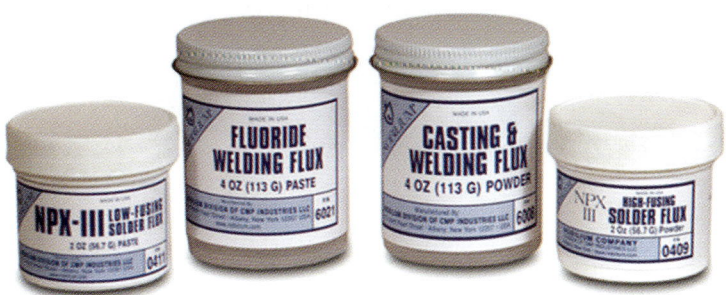

Fig. 75: Soldering fluxes

Plate 42

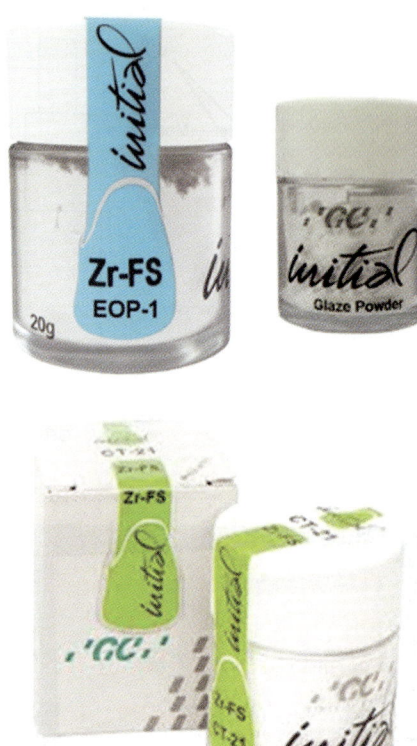

Fig. 76: Ceramic powder of various varieties [enamel, dentin, incisal, cervical (gingival, marginal), glaze, etc.] supplied with special liquid (distilled water).

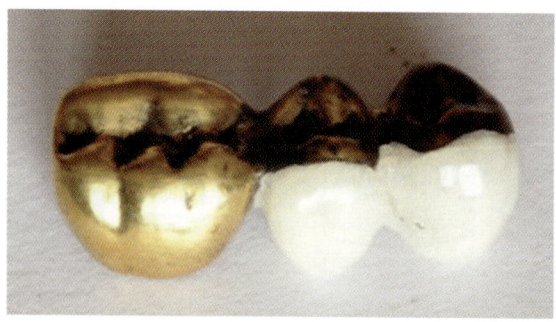

Fig. 77: Metal ceramic restoration (Noble metal alloys)

Plate 43

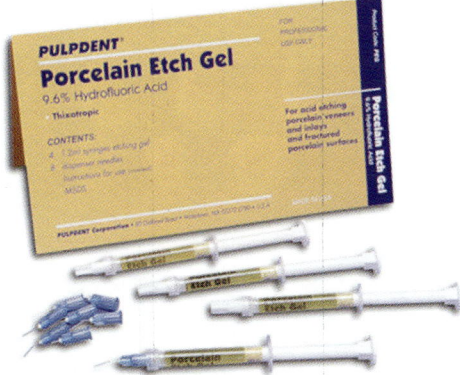

Fig. 77a: Porcelain etch gel containing HF used during cementation to improve mechanical bonding

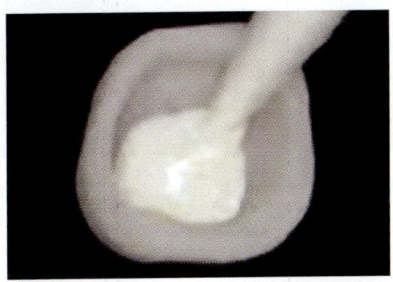

Fig. 77b: preformed polycarbonate crown for cementation

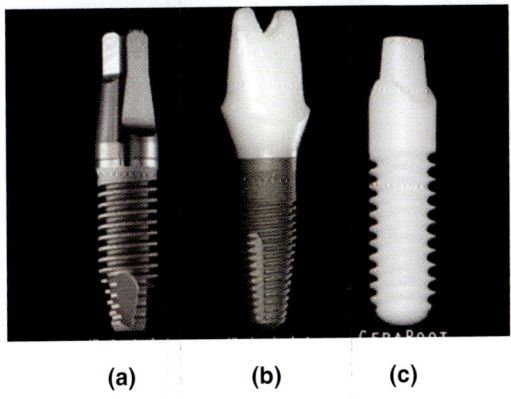

(a)	(b)	(c)

Fig. 78: Titanium implant with titanium abutment coated with hydroxyl apatite (a), Ti implant with Zirconia abutment (b), Zirconia implant (c)

Plate 44

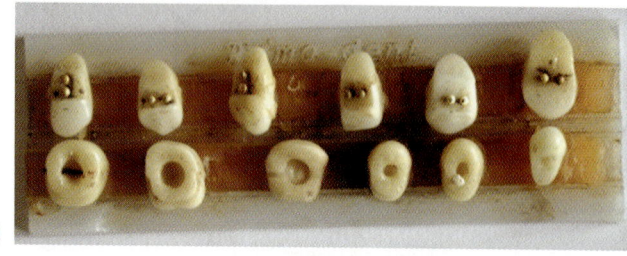

(a)

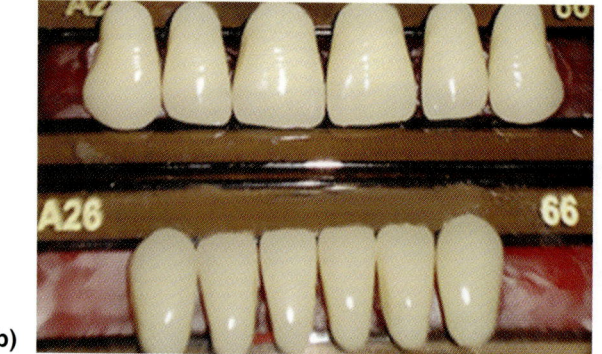

(b)

Fig. 79: (a) Porcelain teeth and (b) acrylic teeth

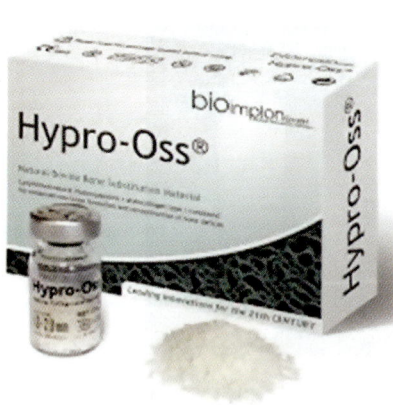

Fig. 80: Hydroxyapatite bone graft material

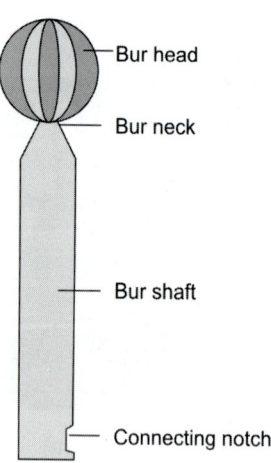

Fig. 81: Parts of dental bur

Plate 45

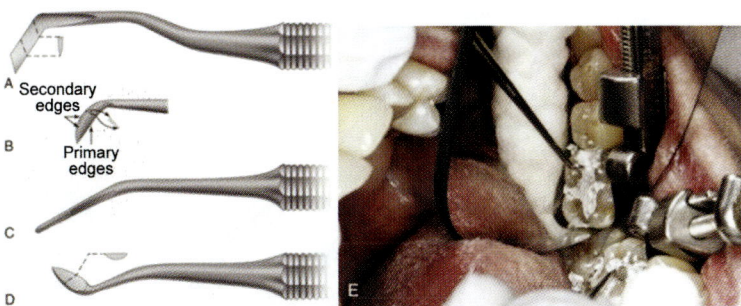

Fig. 82: Hand cutting instruments used for amalgam restoration procedures

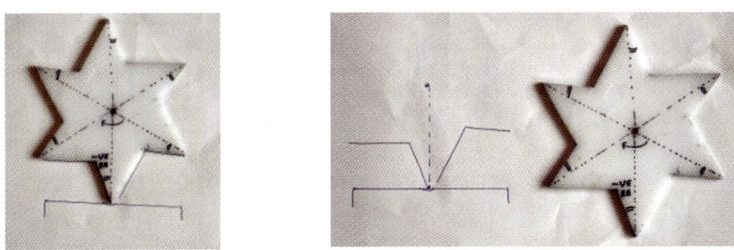

Fig. 83: Cross section of bur

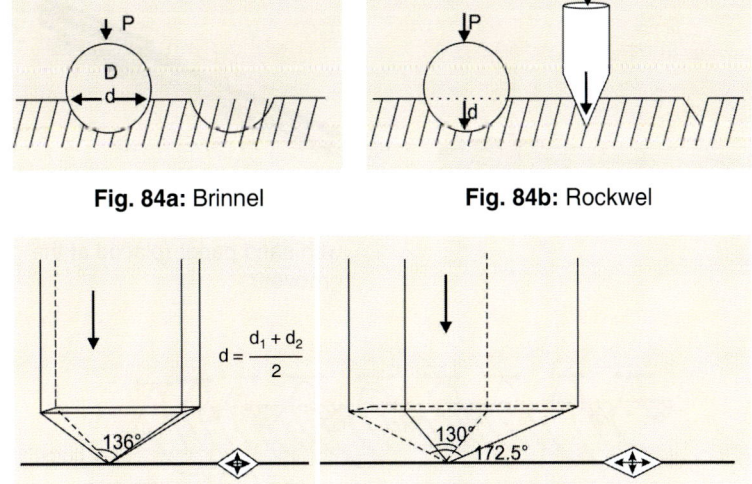

Fig. 84a: Brinnel

Fig. 84b: Rockwel

Fig. 84c: Vicker

Fig. 84d: Knoop

Fig. 84: Surface hardness testing indentor shapes

Plate 46

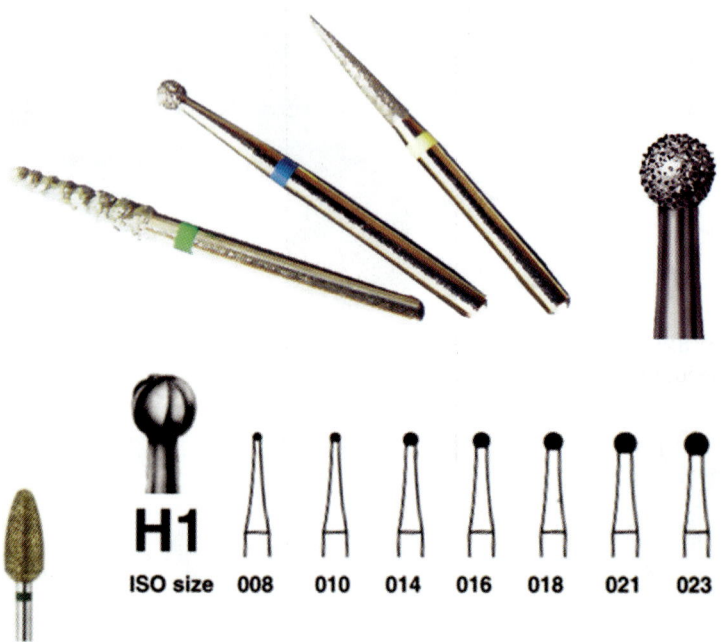

Fig. 85a: Diamond abrasive points

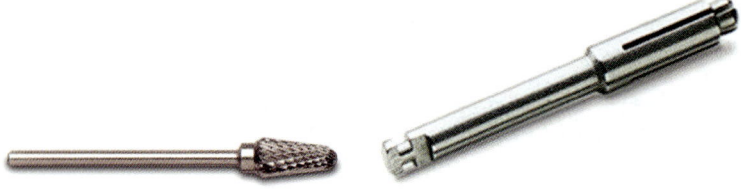

Fig. 85b: Carbide burs

Fig. 85c: Mandrel for polishing with sand paper (placed at the grooves)

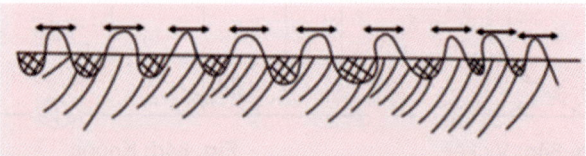

Fig. 86a: Microcrystalline Bielby layer (polished reflecting surface)

Plate 47

Prophy Stone Points

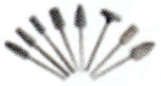 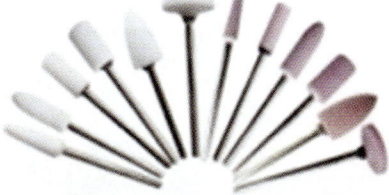
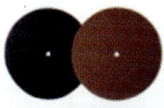

Silicon Cutting Discs

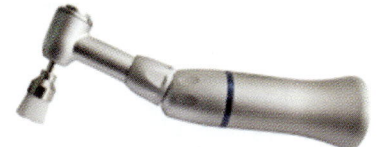

Prophy Brushes

Soft Nylon
Colorful
Cheap price

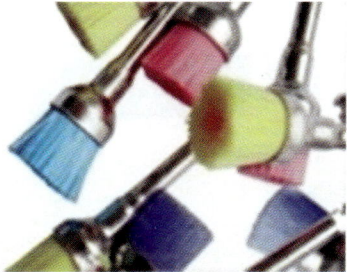

Silicon Wheel/Points

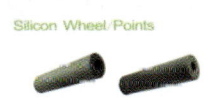 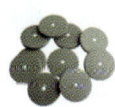 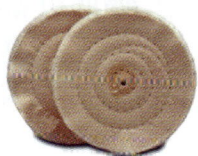

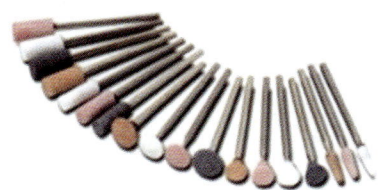 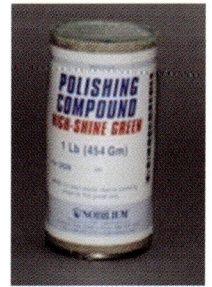

Fig. 86b: Polishing stones, wheels and brushes

Plate 48

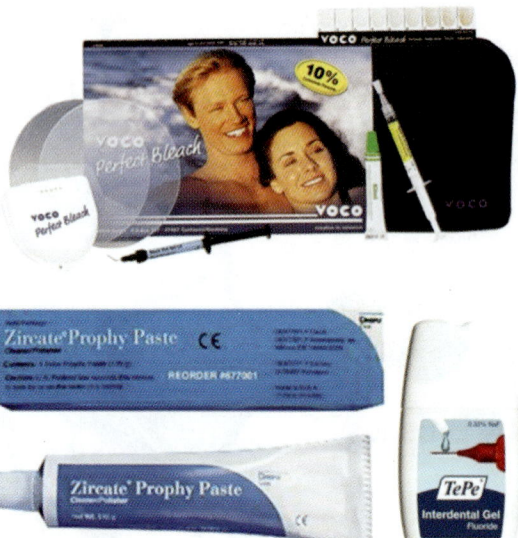

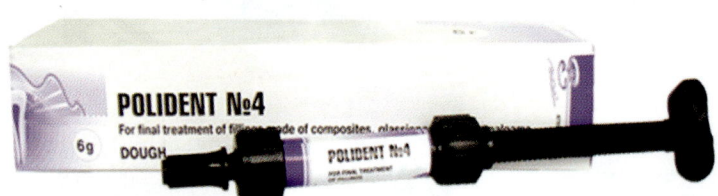

Fig. 87: Polishing dough composite, glass-ionomer and amalgam fillings

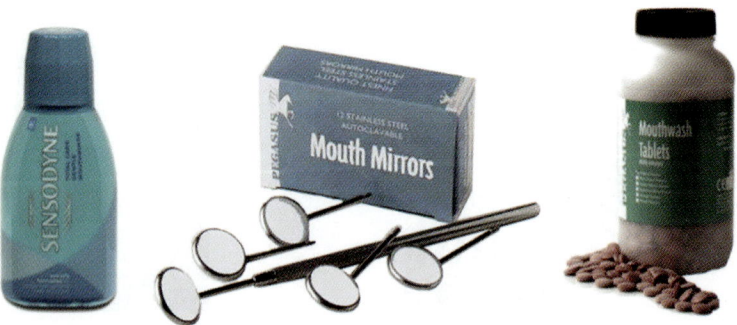

Fig. 88: Mouth mirrors, mouth washes